Vision

Self-Healing

Self-Help

STEPHEN LAU

DEDICATION

This book is dedicated to all
who wish to improve their vision irrespective of their age.

CONTENTS

ONE

BEFORE BEGINNING
VISION SELF-HEALING

WHY YOU ARE HERE

You are here reading this book because you want to improve your vision. Or, maybe, someone has given you a copy of this book, and you are still skeptical, wondering if you can *actually* improve your vision through reading this book.

Rest assured, this book *can* and *will* improve your vision! Honestly, at worst, in the long run, you may still have to wear your corrective lenses, but your vision will not deteriorate any further over the long haul. At best, you may do without your glasses or contact lenses for the rest of your life. This, of course, all depends on YOU! That is, how much effort you are going to put into your vision improvement. Remember, there is no miracle cure. This book only provides all the information you will ever need to achieve your goal in vision improvement.

My purpose in writing this book is to show you that life *can* change for the better if you have the know-how. Right information is powerful. The information in this book is based on my painstaking research on vision health and self-healing, as well as on my own experience. If it works for me and for many, I don't see why it will not work for *you*. Having said that, having the right mindset is equally important, because self-healing begins with the mind *first*, and not with the body. So, empower yourself with everything detailed and outlined in this book. The concise and yet detailed information is written in simple and plain language, presented in a well-organized manner to make it easy for you to understand and to follow. This is a blueprint for long-term vision health and eyesight improvement.

But the information alone will not work miracles for your eyes. It is only the application of the information that will guarantee your success in your vision self-healing endeavor.

Here is the magic formula for your ultimate success in vision self-healing:

- Find out what you *must* do to your eyes.

- Do it accordingly—and co*nsistently* at that!

- Be aware of what you are doing, and make sure it is working for *you*. It is all about *awareness*.

- Do it more often and do it some more!

SELF-HEALING FUNDAMENTALS

In order to heal yourself of any eye problem you may already have, you need to know the fundamentals of self-healing.

- **Intention to heal**

  Life is all about choices. Your life is but the sum of some of the choices—some good, some not so good, and some bad ones—that you have made throughout your life. Intention to heal is one of the choices you have to make in order to be healed. Healing does not take place on its own; it has to be *initiated*.

  Lao Tzu, the famous ancient Chinese philosopher, once said: "A journey of a thousand miles begins with taking the first step." If you want vision self-healing, you must demonstrate your intention to heal yourself. Nobody can make that choice for you, except yourself. Have the intention to heal your vision at all cost!

- **Desire to heal**

  Many people know what to do or rather what they *should* do, but most of them still don't do it; knowing is one thing, while doing it is another. There is always a strong inner voice that smothers the desire and intention to heal. You must overcome that strong inner voice through self-suggestions. (See CHAPTER TWO.)

- **Knowledge to heal**

In order to do something, you need to know *why* you should do it, as well as *how* to do it right. Without such knowledge, you may not even want to do it at all—including *how* to heal yourself. Knowledge takes away your fear to accept the challenge and to confront the outcome of your endeavor.

- **Goals to heal**

There is a saying: "Seeing is believing." But if you "believe" what you "see" in your mind's eye, you will "see" the result of what you "believe"; that is, if you believe what you see, you will see what you believe—this is the power of visualization. To do this, first of all, you must set *goals* to heal yourself, and then *visualize* yourself healed as a result of achieving those goals. Seeing the realization of some of your goals will further reinforce your belief.

- **Commitment to heal**

Like any endeavor, the road to success is often paved with many obstacles and setbacks. To overcome these stumbling blocks, you need commitment, which is practice and practice, and more practice. All natural healing takes time, and nature cannot be rushed. Patience and perseverance hold the key to your success in vision self-healing.

Healing the eye is all about *awareness*. Vision self-healing is about the application of this awareness in your everyday life. It is just that simple!

WHAT TO DO NEXT?

- Read through this entire book to get a general overview of vision health and eyesight improvement. How well you see is the result of how much you have learned to use your eyes through this book.

- Practice what you have learned. Find time and an area to practice vision improvement. Make it an important part of your daily life: if it is only something to fit in with your time, it might never fit in. Make vision improvement one of the top priorities of your daily life! Show yourself that you are serious about vision health and self-healing.

- Develop your eye awareness (See Appendix A.) to constantly remind yourself of what to do and what not to do regarding your vision.

- Reduce the time you wear your eyeglasses or contact lenses. It is important that you make adjustments at home to do your daily chores without your eyeglasses or contacts. It is equally important that you do not strain or squint when you are without them. Get a weaker prescription or wear your old glasses, if need be.

- Find time to spend outdoors without your eyeglasses or contacts.

The bottom line: improve your eyesight as much as possible to reduce, if not totally eliminate, the use of eyeglasses or contacts.

MY OWN STORY

Many years ago, I was afflicted with *myasthenia gravis*, a chronic autoimmune disease affecting the skeletal (voluntary) muscles of the body. The hallmark of *myasthenia gravis* is muscle weakness, which increases during periods of activity and improves after periods of rest. Certain muscles, such as those that control the eyes and eyelid movements, facial expression, talking, chewing and swallowing, are often involved in this disorder. In addition, the muscles that control breathing, neck, and limb movements may also be adversely affected.

One of the main causes of *myasthenia gravis* is stress. I did not know how to relax myself.

One day, I felt intense pressure on my eyes. My first concern was glaucoma (a condition of increased fluid pressure inside the eye). I went to see an ophthalmologist; suspecting that I might be afflicted with *myasthenia gravis*, he immediately referred me to a neurologist, who confirmed the diagnosis after running some medical tests.

According to the diagnosis, I had developed ocular symptoms: ptosis (drooping of eyelids) and diplopia (double vision) in my *myasthenia gravis*. Both of my eyelids drooped, as if my eyes were tired, and I could not open my eyes wide enough to see properly.

My physical conditions also deteriorated rapidly within a

few days. My neck and limb muscles were so weak that I had to use a neck-rest to prop up my head when I was driving; I could hardly use my fingers to control the mouse when I was using my computer; and I could not even raise my hand without having to use the other hand to prop it up.

Fortunately, I did not experience any weakness of the muscles of my pharynx, which could cause difficulty in chewing and swallowing, as well as slurred speech—symptoms not uncommon in *myasthenia gravis*.

At first, I was prescribed pyridostigmine (mestinon) as the usual first-line treatment for my immune disorder.

After several months, my conditions did not improve. I was given another prescription, prednisone, a synthetic hormone commonly referred to as a "steroid," for my *myasthenia gravis*. Prednisone acts as a long-term immunosuppressant to control the production of antibodies. Essentially, it serves to stabilize my so-called "overactive" immune system.

The adverse side effects of prednisone for my *myasthenia gravis* included decreased resistance to infection, indigestion, hypertension, weight gain, swelling of the face, thinning of skin, predisposition to osteoporosis, and potential development of cataracts and glaucoma. The long list was not only depressing but also frightening. I was worried that I would have to take my medications for the rest of my life, not just for my *myasthenia gravis* but also for the many side effects related to the drugs, such as bone loss, weight gain, and high blood pressure, among others.

Initially, after several months on steroid medications, there was some improvement in the symptoms, but overall it was neither significant nor encouraging. Specifically, my eyelids no longer drooped, but the right eye and the left eye did not align (my right eye being much stronger than my left eye), and therefore resulting in double vision.

7

After almost two years on prednisone, my neurologist, seeing there was little improvement in my *myasthenia gravis*, switched me to azathioprine, a drug supposedly with fewer side effects. However, that medication did not seem to have any positive effect on my symptoms, let alone my double vision. Naturally, I became frustrated.

Now, when I look back at the whole episode, I would think that my illness might have been a blessing in disguise. Everything happens in one's life with a divine purpose. In many ways, I was grateful that I had the illness—which has changed my life forever and for the better. I began to learn how to take care of my health, and I knew I had to do it on my own.

I was in a dilemma: on the one hand, I needed improvement in my neuromuscular transmission to increase my muscle strength and to eliminate my double vision; on the other hand, I knew that if *myasthenia gravis* did not kill me, the many side effects of the medications might eventually undo me.

I made a decision to change drastically my diet, accompanied by a regular fast, in an attempt to discontinue all my medications ultimately. The initial results were encouraging. Instead of gaining weight, I had lost more than fifteen pounds; instead of jacking up my blood pressure, I had made it plummet. I had won my initial battle against all the adverse side effects of medications for my *myasthenia gravis*. I knew that I had to do *more*—much more than that. My rude awakening finally came: there was no miracle cure for my *myasthenia gravis*; only my wholesome wellness would bring about recovery and natural self-healing.

Slowly and gradually, I discontinued *all* my medications. Finally, I did it! Now, I am 100 percent drug free!

To eliminate double vision, the doctor recommended wearing an eye-patch over my weaker eye. But I did not entertain the idea of wearing an eye-patch—looking like a pirate of the Caribbean Sea. Besides, wearing an eye-patch would not solve my problem of double vision. There is a Chinese saying: "Cut your toes to avoid the worms." I thought that was precisely what the doctor recommended: getting around the problem instead of solving it. I also recalled that early on, when my muscles were weak and I asked him for recommended remedy, he told me not to use those weak muscles. I disagreed with the doctor; instead, I exercised my weaker muscles until they became much stronger.

That was how I began my journey of self-healing.

Now, more than two decades later, I am 100 percent drug free.

Having said that, my *myasthenia gravis* symptoms sometimes recur, but they are not as serious as they were when I was under prescribed medications more than two decades ago. Every now and then, I do feel *strain* in my eyes—I understand that has to do with my eye muscle, which are being constantly used. The only thing I can do is to relax my eyes regularly. Over the years, my vision has deteriorated, partly due to the constant eye strain and partly due to the progressive aging of the eyes.

After years of research, I came up with a book, **My Myasthenia Gravis**, describing how I have learned to cope with my autoimmune disease. The doctor told me that there was no cure for an autoimmune disease, Maybe there is no *complete* cure, but one can learn to cope with the disease symptoms and eliminate as many of them without the use of prescription drugs. By the same token, you can also significantly improve your vision despite the vision problems you may already have through eye aging,

Remember, nothing is set in stone, and you can always reverse your current eye conditions if you set your mind to it.

Just believe in yourself, and do what you can with what you have and let God do the rest.

TWO

VISION: A MATTER OF THE MIND

THE MIND TO HEAL

Vision is a matter of the mind, not just the eye.

Vision self-healing, like any other healing, begins with the mind *first*, and not the body or the eye for that matter.

The *intention* to heal comes from within, specifically, the mind. With intention, comes *concentration* and then *focus* to empower yourself with the knowledge to heal your eyes of any vision problem you may have. The manifestation of the mind is reflected throughout the healing process.

Healing begins with the mind, and mind healing is always mind over matter.

Changing for the Better

The mind can either heal or harm. Your mind can help you improve your vision because vision healing is all in the mind, but it can also increase your subconscious internal resistance to following new patterns requisite for self-healing.

All vision begins with thoughts. Seeing is a matter of the mind. To see better, you need to *change* not only the way you "think" about seeing but also the way you "go about" seeing. It is all in the mind—*your* thinking mind!

Changing your **vision habits**, most of which may be incorrect or even damaging to your vision health, is not an easy task. Once these visual patterns are deeply ingrained in your mind, they have become your long-term memories, and to change them or to eradicate them becomes a new challenge. But you can and you must overcome that challenge through your mind power.

Harness your mind power to do two things for you:

- To restore your memories of clear, sharp visual images

- To visualize familiar images of clear vision, such as imagining total darkness in order to totally relax your optic nerve (total relaxation occurring only in total darkness) connected to your brain.

Memory and imagination are powerful tools for you to improve your vision, because your mind has a deep connection with your eyes. Effectively using your mind can successfully stimulate clearer and better vision. It is always mind over matter.

Changing vision habits

How do you change your bad vision habits? There is a saying: "It is difficult to teach an old dog new tricks." The conscious mind is often reluctant and resistant to any change. Believe it or not, most of us are stubborn creatures—more like an old dog—who do not want to get out of own comfort zones. The only way to overcome this obstacle is through changing the subconscious mind.

Basically, your mind is made up of your conscious mind and your subconscious mind. Your conscious mind makes decisions and you act accordingly, but it is your subconscious mind that directs your conscious mind. That is to say, in your conscious mind, you are fully aware of your actions and their respective consequences; in your subconscious mind, where you store your emotions and memories, you only respond *spontaneously* to repetitions of words and images in the form of affirmations and visualization. In other words, if you keep on repeating positive self-suggestions or visualizing positive images in your mind's eye, you *can* effectively change the thoughts in your conscious mind through your subconscious mind.

Affirmations and visualization

To initiate any meaningful change, you must rely on your mind, specifically, your subconscious mind. Give your mind the tools it needs to change for the better.

Your thoughts pre-determine how your eyes function. Use positive affirmations and creative images to *change* your thinking in order to change *how* your eyes should function.

Affirmations and visualization are powerful mind-power tools to change your subconscious mind in order to change your conscious mind. They are effective in changing your bad vision habits that inhibit vision self-healing. Remember, these bad vision habits may have become long-term memories in your subconscious mind. You must eradicate them!

Creating your affirmations

For affirmations or self-suggestions to be effective, they must meet the following criteria:

- They must be simple and easy to remember (Always use the **present tense**!).

- They must be practical, realistic, and achievable. (Do not visualize yourself as a billionaire!)

- They must be what you strongly believe in, not just what you wish for. (Always know the difference between what you need and what you want!)

- They must be repeatedly constantly and consistently in order to have an impact on your subconscious mind. (Always be consistent and persistent!)

You can repeat to yourself daily the following positive affirmations or self-suggestions (of course, you can always make up your own self-suggestions):

- I am willing to accept any change in order to heal my eyes.

- I am learning how to correct my bad vision habits in order to see better.

- I am working diligently to achieve my goal in vision self-healing.

- I am committed to improving my vision.

- I believe one day I do not have to wear glasses.

- I possess the mind power to overcome any challenge in my pursuit of vision self-healing.

Creating your visualization

Visualization is the use of positive images to create the "reality" in your subconscious mind such that "seeing" the positive result of your efforts reinforces your determination and perseverance to reach your goal of vision self-healing.

Visualization plays a pivotal part in your vision improvement: you visualize *what* your eyes can see through your efforts, as well as *how* your eyes can improve through regular practice.

Vision research has attested to the close connection between the mind (visualization) and vision (focusing). If you visualize seeing a distant object, the focusing mechanism of your eye can physically respond to your imagination; that is, your eye can actually *change* its focus through visualization.

In visualization, you close your eyes in your imagination, you relax them in your imagination, and then you re-open them in your imagination. It is all in your imagination.

Awareness to avoid eyestrain

Develop your mental awareness to change your bad vision habits that cause eyestrain.

- **Shifting**: Train your mind to *edge* or *trace* the outline of any visual object with your eyes. Form this good vision habit to avoid "staring" or "eye fixation."

- **Eye balancing**: Wear an eye-patch (obtainable at a pharmacy or local drug store) over your stronger eye in order to strengthen your weaker eye.

- **Periphery**: Use a two-eyed patch to cover your eyes to enhance your peripheral vision. Make a two-eyed patch out of a strip of stiff cardboard (3" x 1"), with a small part cut off in the middle to accommodate your nose.

- **Sunglasses**: Avoid wearing sunglasses to avoid "squinting."

MIND RELAXATION

The eye conditions are constantly changing such that they can be adversely affected by any emotional or mental stress, resulting in **eyestrain** that can cause vision blur. By the same token, you can significantly improve your vision if you relax your eyes completely through relaxation

Using a Relaxed Mind to Relax the Body

It is almost impossible to relax just your eyes, while the rest of your body remains tense and stressed. Total relaxation begins with the mind *first*, and then the rest of the body, including the eyes. Use your mind to relax your body, and then your eyes. The best way to achieve mental relaxation is by *meditation*.

Meditation to relax the mind

Meditation is a proven mind-body therapy for body-mind relaxation.

The healing power of meditation lies in its capability to focus the mind solely on the very *present moment*, thereby removing memories of the past and worries of the future. Meditation helps you focus your mind on the present moment to the exclusion of past and future thoughts. The mind in its natural and perfect stillness relaxes completely.

In contemporary living, your mind is often riddled with thoughts of what you just did, what you will do, or should have done. Nearly all your thoughts, including your desires and fears, are based on either the past or the future. Your desires are no more than recollections of the past pleasures and hopes of repeating them in the future. Fears are also memories of past pain, and your efforts to avoid the pain in the future. All these rambling thoughts in your subconscious mind indirectly affect your conscious mind, and hence your body and your eyes.

In the present, your mind is always preoccupied with the past or the future, leaving little or no room for the present moment, which, ironically enough, is the *only* reality. The past was gone, and the future is unknown; only the present is "real." The present is a gift, and that is why it is called "present." But, unfortunately, most of us do not live in the present, not to mention appreciate it, because the present is interlaced with the past and the future. Meditation is about re-focusing on the present moment.

The mental focus of meditation is not quite the same as the mental concentration, such as solving a difficult math problem or while performing a complex mental task. Meditation is focusing on something seemingly *insignificant* (such as your breathing) or *spontaneous* (such as eating and even driving) such that your mind can be conditioned to focusing on only the present moment. In this way, your mind concentration excludes all past and future thoughts, thereby instrumental in giving your mind a meaningful break. It is in this sublime mental state that you are capable of understanding the true nature of things, and their relativity to the meaning of life and existence. Meditation awakens you to what is real or what is *quasi* real.

Points to remember when you meditate:

- Focus on an *object* as your focal point of concentration: your own breathing; looking at a candle flame; listening to a sound (such as the sound of running water from a fountain); watching your footsteps when you are walking, or just about *anything* that can easily draw you back to your meditation.

- Palming is an excellent exercise not just for vision improvement, but also for deep meditation. (See **palming exercise** in CHAPTER FIVE.)

- During your meditation, if your mind wanders away (which is quite common), gently direct your mind to re-focus on the same object of your concentration. Learn how to focus through your act of *noticing* that your mind has wandered off, as well as through your repetitive efforts. Meditation is all about focusing on the present moment. Make focusing a habit of relaxation for your eyes

- Keep yourself in *full consciousness*: you must be fully aware of what is going on around you. That explains why in meditation (except in the walking meditation) you need to sit erect in order to keep your body in full consciousness. Do not lie down (or else you may fall asleep); do not slouch (this may not help you focus).

A full *lotus position* is not required. However, it is important that you maintain a *consistent* position or posture with your thumb tip and forefinger tip of each hand touching very lightly, while the other fingers are either curled or extended out. A consistent posture and hand position will promote a *meditative mind* to practice your meditation techniques.

Breathing right to relax and to meditate

Breathing is important in meditation because it is the focal point of the mind. In addition, breathing out is associated with "letting go" and "body detoxification"— essential components to relax the body and the mind.

In meditation, focus on your natural breath as it flows in and out. Notice how you inhale and exhale. You will begin to feel yourself becoming relaxed and soothed.

Diaphragm breathing

Diaphragm breathing is the complete breath. Consciously change your breathing pattern. Use your diaphragm to breathe (the diaphragm muscle separating your chest from your abdomen). If you place one hand on your breastbone, feeling that it is raised, with the other hand above your waist, feeling the diaphragm muscle moving up and down, then you are practicing diaphragm breathing correctly. Deep breathing with your diaphragm gives you complete breath.

This is *how* you do diaphragm breathing:

- Sit comfortably.

- Begin your slow exhalation through your nose.

- Contract your abdomen to empty your lungs.

- Begin your slow inhalation and *simultaneously* make your belly bulge out.

- Continuing your slow inhalation, now, slightly contract your abdomen and simultaneously lift your chest and hold.

- Continue your slow inhalation, and slowly raise your shoulders. This allows the air to enter fully your lungs to attain the complete breath.

- Retain your breath with your shoulders slightly raised for a count of 5.

- Very slowly exhale the air.

- Repeat the process.

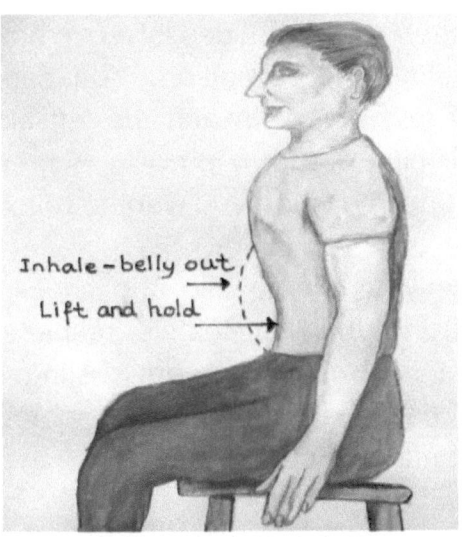

Inhale – belly out,

Lift and hold

Diaphragm Breathing

Learn to slowly prolong your breath, especially your exhalation. Relax your chest and diaphragm muscle, so that you can extend your exhalation, making your breathing out complete.

To prolong your exhalation, count "one-and-two-and-three" as you breathe in and breathe out. Make sure that they become balanced. Once you have mastered that, then try to make your breathing out a little longer than your breathing in.

Alternate-nostril breathing

Alternate-nostril breathing is a basic Yoga breathing exercise to balance the right side and the left side of your brain.

The left side of your brain governs the right side of your body, including your speech and logical thinking, while the right side of your brain governs the left side of your body, including your creativity and intuition. Achieving balance and harmony between the two sides of your brain is critical to mind healing for deep relaxation. You can balance your mental energy from the right and the left side of the brain through practicing alternate-nostril breathing during meditation, or anytime when you want to relax your eyes.

- Place your thumb and ring finger lightly on your right and your left nostrils, respectively, with your index and middle fingers resting lightly on your forehead between your eyebrows. (See the illustration below)

- Exhale deeply through both nostrils.

- Press your thumb against the RIGHT nostril to CLOSE it.

- Breathe in through your LEFT nostril. Count 8.

- CLOSE your LEFT nostril by pressing down your ring finger. Now, both nostrils are closed. Retain the air, and count 4.

- OPEN your RIGHT nostril, and breathe out. Count 8.

- With the LEFT nostril still CLOSED, breathe in through the RIGHT nostril. Count 8.

- CLOSE the RIGHT nostril. Now, both nostrils are closed. Retain the air, and count 4

- OPEN the LEFT nostril, and breathe out with the RIGHT nostril still closed. Count 8

- Repeat the above process.

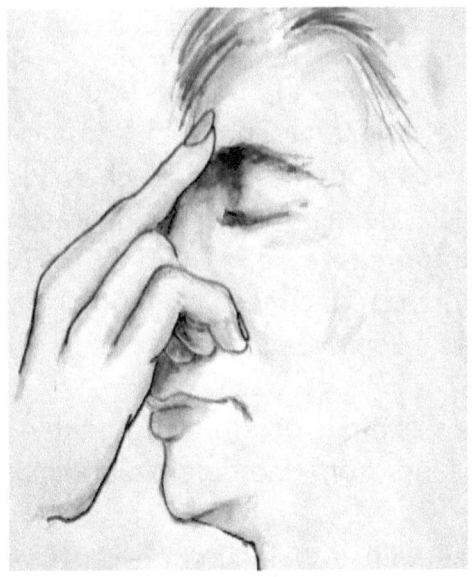

Alternate-Nostril Breathing

Here is a summary of alternate-nostril breathing:

- Breathe out through BOTH nostrils.

- Breathe in through the LEFT nostril (count 8).

- Close BOTH nostrils, and retain air (count 4).

- Breathe out through the RIGHT nostril (count 8).

- Breathe in through the RIGHT nostril (count 8).

- Close BOTH nostrils, and retain air (count 4).

- Breathe out through the LEFT nostril (count 8).

- Repeat.

Using the Mind to Relax the Eyes

The eyes are active throughout your waking hours. As a result, they are constantly in strain and stress. They do not know how to relax, unless they receive direct instructions from your conscious mind, or when they are in *total darkness* (see **eye palming exercise** in <u>CHAPTER FIVE</u>).

Constantly, you unconsciously strain and stress your eyes under the following eye conditions:

- Eyes fixating or staring (healthy eyes constantly "shifting" from one detail to another)

- Eyes with unbalanced vision (i.e. one eye being much stronger than the other one, for example, lazy eye)

- Eyes using only their central vision to see, while neglecting their peripheral vision, resulting in restricted vision field (healthy eyes see with both *central vision* and *peripheral vision*)

- Eyes squinting from "excess" light (healthy eyes easily adapting and adjusting to light)

Use the mind to correct the above eye conditions that cause constant eyestrain damaging to vision health.

THREE

VISION AWARENESS
AND
EYE DISORDERS

THE HUMAN EYE

The human eye is not just a mechanical tool for vision; it is one of the body's most important body organs. The importance of the human eye is due to the following:

- It gives perception and vision of the outside world. Eyesight is the most important of your five senses.

- It is also connected to the inner world—your mind. Seeing is believing, and perception is reality. Your vision affects your perception, and hence your personality; it creates your own world.

- It is inter-connected with different body organs, such as the brain (which controls *how* you see), the heart (which pumps blood and transports oxygen to your eyes), the liver (which supplies nutrients to the eye, according to Chinese medicine).

How the Eye Functions

Simply put, you cannot see without *light*.

- When you see an object, the light from that object passes through the **lens** (in front of the eyeball), which is held in place by **ciliary muscles** in your eye.

- The lens then focuses the image on the **retina** (at the back of the eyeball), which sends the visual information through the **optic nerve** to the brain.

The human lens is designed for distant vision, not close vision. When the object is too close (i.e. less than 20 feet away), the ciliary muscles must contract in order to focus the visual image *correctly* on the retina. This process of contraction or expansion of the eye muscles is known as **accommodation**.

AWARENESS Consciously train your eyes for distant vision! Regularly look up from your computer or your book!

How the Eye Malfunctions

Poor vision is a result of the malfunctioning of the human eye, causing all types of vision problems.

- When the ciliary muscles are too weak to contract properly, the focal image of a *distant* object may fall *in front of* the retina (i.e. when the eyeball is *too long*), instead of directly *on* the retina itself, and hence it creates a blurred image. This happens in **nearsightedness**.

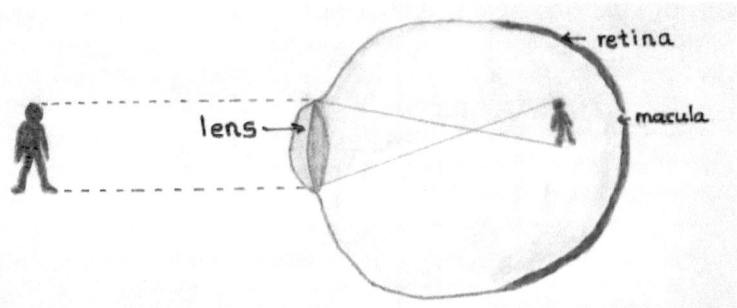

- When the ciliary muscles are too weak to contract properly, the focal image of a *close* object may fall *beyond* the retina (i.e. when the eyeball is *too short*), the resulting visual image becomes blurry and distorted. This happens in **farsightedness**.

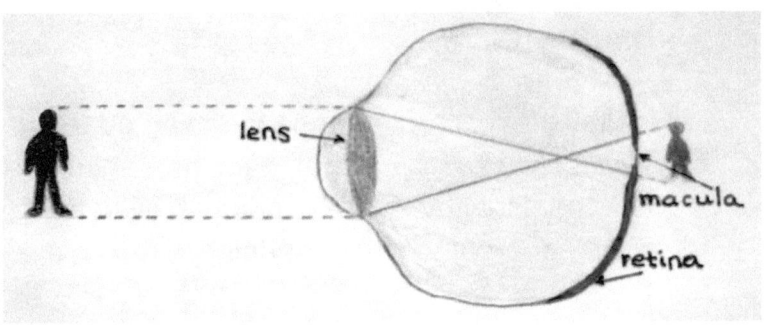

The main causes of eye malfunctioning are:

- Mental stress

- Eye muscle strain.

Therefore, the key to vision self-healing is to address these two critical issues.

AWARENESS: The shape of the eyeball determines the power of vision. The relaxation level of the eye pre-determines the shape of the eyeball.

HEALTHY VISION

Vision is about the eye. It is all about what you see, or how well you see. Healthy vision gives you *sensation*, *perception*, and *conception*. Your life depends on your eyes. In short, healthy vision gives you all the raw materials for living for life.

Vision is *seeing*, which involves not just the eyes, but also the mind, and the brain as well.

- Healthy vision requires healthy eyes with healthy light-sensing cells to receive and process visual information.

- Healthy vision requires a health mind so that it can *selectively see* the visual data presented before the eyes. Healthy eyes do not see *everything*, nor do they *attempt* to see everything.

  AWARENESS: See only *selectively*! Never STRAIN your eyes to see! A blurry image is OK!

- Healthy vision requires a healthy brain to *interpret correctly* the visual data selectively collected by the eye.

Therefore, healthy vision is a complex interaction between the eye, the mind, and the brain. The physical body (specifically, the physical and physiological health) and the environment (such as lighting) can positively or negatively influence this complex interaction between the eye, the mind, and the brain. In other words, vision health is *holistic* health. Accordingly, vision self-healing cannot address only the human eye alone; as a matter of fact, vision self-healing begins with the mind *first*, and then the eye, and the body.

To conclude, healthy vision is a balance and correlation of physical eyesight, emotional seeing, and inner vision.

How to have better visual images

- **Good lighting** to stimulate the light-sensing cells of your eyes (millions of light-sensing cells in the retina)

- **Relaxed ciliary muscles** to hold the lens in its proper place

- **Relaxed eyeballs** to retain their shape

- A **relaxed macula** (near the center of the retina) to prevent intense use of central vision, or staring, causing eyestrain

- A **relaxed mind** to correctly interpret and process the visual data received

Good vision is all about **relaxation**.

POOR VISION

Poor vision is lack of clarity when seeing near or far away. Poor vision creates vision problems, such as *nearsightedness* (typical in younger people) and *farsightedness* (typical in older people).

Both of these weak or impaired eye conditions are due to mental stress and eye muscle fatigue.

Nearsightedness

Nearsightedness (also known as **myopia**) is the inability to see *distant* objects clearly. This eye condition tends to develop in younger people, especially young children.

Nearsightedness in children may be due to the following:

- Initial fascination with wearing eyeglasses

- Boredom with learning (a blurry mind leading to blurry vision—an example of how the mind can affect vision)

- Too many near-focusing tasks or activities (e.g. computer vision syndrome or video games)

- Formation of bad vision habits

Nearsightedness may have many adverse complications. Once myopia (nearsightedness) worsens, more serious eye problems and disorders can potentially develop, including the following:

- **Cataracts** (cloudy lenses)

- **Detached retina** (loosening of the light receptive layer at the back of the eye)

- **Glaucoma** (increased pressure stressing the optic nerve)

- **Macular degeneration** (impaired central vision due to disease or aging)

Farsightedness

Farsightedness (also known as **hyperopia**) is the inability to see *close* objects clearly. This condition tends to develop in older people in their forties and fifties due to the following:

- Mental stress (divorces, relationship problems, financial stress, retirement etc.)

- Years of lifestyle abuse (e.g. drugs, drinking, and smoking)

- Accumulation of bad vision habits over the years

How Vision Deteriorates

Conventional curative eye-care is damaging to the eye

because it focuses on prescribing corrective eyeglasses or contacts for artificially clear sight. Unfortunately, at worst, eyeglasses or contacts do more harm to the eye; at best, they never improve vision to normal.

The explanation is that constantly wearing corrective lenses will constantly maintain the eye's **refractive error**, and thus leading to the steady increase of the strength of the corrective lenses in order to maintain the same visual acuity. In other words, wearing eyeglasses or contacts only makes vision worse, and not better, because it makes you subconsciously crave for clear vision. In order to see better, you strain your eyes, and eyestrain only leads to further vision deterioration. Before long, you need another pair of corrective eyeglasses with a stronger prescription. This is *how* your vision goes from bad to worse. Ask yourself how many pairs of eyeglasses you have obtained for yourself over the years, with each pair having a stronger prescription than the previous one.

The truth of the matter" corrective lenses only perpetuate the eye's refractive errors.

- They are only "crutches" for artificially clear eyesight; they do not correct poor vision.

- They do not accurately reflect your eye conditions, which change constantly, from moment to moment, according to the physical environment and your mental conditions.

- They do not let your eyes adapt naturally to the mind; in other words, they disconnect the eye from the mind.

- They perpetuate the refractive error of your eyes, leading to more eyestrain and ultimately stronger prescriptions.

AWARENESS: No need to go for perfect vision! Never **strain** your eyes in order to see better!

Poor vision leads to further vision loss and impairment, resulting in **legal blindness** (20 percent or less vision), which is defined as 20/200, that is, the capability of seeing within 20 feet what a person with normal vision can see within 200 feet. Legal blindness occurs to more than 10 percent of population aged between 50 to 69, and more than 70 percent aged 70 and over.

Wearing contact lenses is not any better than wearing eyeglasses. As a matter of fact, wearing contacts may have many other less-than-desirable side effects:

- Distortion of the cornea

- Drying out of the eye

- Eye infection and inflammation

- Irritation of the eye and eyelids

- Oxygen deprivation

- Pain and dizziness

- Vision Loss

Laser eye clinics are touting the risks of **laser eye surgery** as minimal, and testimonials of those who have undergone such a surgery attest to the success of this virtually risk-free procedure. The fact of the matter is that 10 percent of laser eye surgeries have complications, and, more importantly, the long-term consequences of the surgery still remain relatively unknown because it is a fairly new procedure on the eye.

The good news is that poor vision loss does not have to be an inevitable consequence of aging. You can successfully improve your vision at any age.

SOME COMMON EYE DISORDERS

Eye disorders, like any disease, often start at the **cellular level** in which oxidation occurs. Cells make up your organs. When cells die, your organs fail and heath deteriorates, and you age and die. The cell of an organ can be destroyed during the process of oxidation in which unpaired electrons, known as **free radicals**, are produced. Free radicals occur naturally as byproducts of oxidation, such as during respiration and other chemical processes; for example, during breathing, while life-giving oxygen is produced, harmful carbon dioxide is also released.

Likewise, eye disorders are related to free radicals and oxidation. According to research studies, oxidation is involved in the development of most eye disorders, including cataracts, retinal disease, and glaucoma.

Macular Degeneration

Often called AMD or ARMD (age-related macular degeneration), macular degeneration is the leading cause of vision loss and blindness in Americans aged 65 and older.

AMD is a degenerative condition of the macula, the part

of the retina responsible for the sharp, central vision needed to read or drive. Because AMD affects the macula, you may lose your central vision or reading vision.

The risk factors

The risk factors for macular degeneration are:

- **Age over 65** with risk increasing proportionately with age

- A **smoker** with 2.5 times increased risk than a non-smoker

- Having **blue eyes** instead of brown eyes (blue eyes enabling the blue-violet sunrays to penetrate deeper into the eye tissues of the retina, and hence a greater chance of developing macular degeneration)

- A **sun worshiper** spending much time outdoors

Given that macular degeneration begins much earlier, from youth through the age of 30 years, deterioration accelerates as aging progresses.

The symptoms

Macular degeneration symptoms include the following:

- Outlines of objects becoming blurry and wavy

- Straight lines becoming crooked; shapes of objects becoming indistinct and steamy

- Much slower reading speed

- A prolonged period of time to adapt when going indoors from a bright outdoor environment

- Eye examination indicating many solar-aging spots on the retina

The treatment

There is little or no cure once the onset of macular degeneration begins. You can retard it, but there is no cure. Prevention is better than no cure. The key to retina health is to keep the retinal blood vessels open, to avoid buildup of cholesterol, blood clots, and calcification.

Laser treatment can arrest the fast-progressing form of macular degeneration, but does not improve vision or preserve eyesight. Therefore, prevention is always the best option.

Eye nutrition can protect the retina from further damage or deterioration.

- **Vitamins A**, **C**, and **E**, and **beta carotene**, which is a precursor for vitamin A, can reduce the risk of developing macular degeneration. It is therefore important that as you grow older you need mega-doses of nutrients because of poor absorption due to inadequate digestive juices for digestion and absorption.

- **Zinc** can retard the loss of protective melanin pigment of the retina against sunlight damage. In addition, zinc helps the release of vitamin A from the liver. Zinc is an important co-factor in getting vitamin A to the retina. However, it must be understood that zinc in excess of 25 milligrams may lead to deficiency of copper, elevation of LDL (bad cholesterol) levels, cholesterol imbalance— all these may cause further damage to the retina. Adequate zinc, but not too much, enhances the retina health.

- **Glutathione** is another powerful antioxidant to protect retinal cells from ultra-violet-A and ultra-violet-B damage. **Selenium** and **riboflavin** stimulate the production of glutathione.

- **Omega-3 fats** can improve vision. However, because they can also cause lipid peroxidation (that is, they turn rancid on exposure to sunlight), you need more antioxidants.

- Nutrition should also include **bioflavonoids**, which are plant pigments with protective properties against sunlight damage. Foods that are rich in bioflavonoids include red onions, red grapes, cherries, and citrus fruits.

In short, your diet plays a pivotal role in retina health, and hence the prevention of macular degeneration.

In addition to diet, give up **nicotine** totally. Reduce your daily intake of caffeine—if you must drink coffee—because it not only interrupts with retinal blood flow but also increases blood pressure, which is bad for the retina.

Aspirin is a blood thinner. It may benefit blood vessel diseases and prevents blockages of oxygen to the brain. However, too much aspirin may also cause retinal bleeding, which impairs retinal health.

Macular degeneration is an eye disease that can be prevented—or at least deferred if you live a healthy lifestyle. Aging is not the cause of degeneration. Retinal disease is a result of accumulative damage to the retina due to neglect, or abuse, or both.

Glaucoma

Glaucoma, another major cause of blindness, is a condition due to increased eye pressure. In conventional medicine, most eye doctors would recommend surgeries and eye drops to relieve high ocular pressure in the eye.

However, there is one problem: surgeries and eye drops would also create a *chronic* condition, ironically enough, leading to ultimate blindness. The use of eye drops may have adverse long-term effects, one of which is the falling off of pieces of iris, causing blockage, and thereby instrumental in increasing eye pressure over the long haul, instead of reducing the eye pressure.

Dr. Leslie Salov, M.D., O.D. Ph.D., in his book *Secrets for Better Vision*, states that most glaucoma patients are highly intelligent professionals who lead very stressful, busy lives. This finding led Dr. Salov to believe that to improve vision or eye health, you need to improve the health of your *entire* person simultaneously because your body is a set of interlocking systems that affect one another. Given that the whole is greater than the sum of its parts, your eyes are only a small part of your whole person. Accordingly, to heal the eyes, you must heal the body *first*. It is just that simple!

To have healthy vision, even as you age, you must employ not only the sciences of physiology, biology, and chemistry, but also the healing powers of philosophy and even spirituality. This is no exception when it comes to treating glaucoma. In other words, to treat glaucoma, you need to examine not just your eyes, but also every aspect of your life, including your emotional and spiritual health.

The methods of glaucoma treatment recommended by Dr. Salov include the following:

- **Visualization** is the use of guided imagery to direct blood, oxygen, and leukocytes (immunity cells) to the eye through a mental image of a healthy eye. Essentially, your conscious mind controls the involuntary processes that occur automatically inside your body. Specifically, visualization relaxes the muscles in the walls of your canal of Schlemm (circular channel in the eye that collects watery substance between the lens and the cornea). By relaxing these muscles, extra fluid can be excreted to relieve the glaucoma pressure. Without using eye drops with chemicals, visualization can naturally relax eye muscles so that your pupils become small enough to open up the canal of Schlemm to excrete the fluid for eye pressure relief.

  However, it must be pointed out that visualization works only when you use it with dedication and consistency. In other words, you have to practice visualization daily and diligently.

- **Meditation** is the art of thinking of nothing to remove everyday stresses and worries. When you are under stress, you body produces chemical changes within your body, which decrease blood flow and oxygen level to your eye. Practice meditation to de-stress yourself. (See **meditation** in <u>CHAPTER TWO</u>.)

Cataracts

About 50 percent of Americans aged 65 and over develop cataracts.

In the normal eye, light passes through the clear lens and is focused on the retina of the eye. In cataracts, the lens becomes cloudy, resulting in opacity that distorts the light rays or prevents the light from focusing on the retina.

The causes

Cataracts are due to the following:

- The lens has become less resilient. The fibers in the lens become compressed and consequently rigid.

- The lens has become less transparent due to the aging process. The lens, made up of protein and water, becomes cloudy due to the coagulation of eye protein.

- The lens has become thicker. The accumulation of deposits of calcium and cholesterol in the lens becomes denser, especially in the center of the lens.

The development of cataracts has nothing to do with the overuse of the eye. Rather, it has to do with the following:

- Alcohol consumption

- Nicotine

- Heredity

- Health problems, such as diabetes

- Medications, such as corticosteroids

- Long-term sun exposure (ultraviolet-A and ultraviolet-B rays)

- Eye injuries

The symptoms

Initially, cataracts do not affect vision much. Then, slowly and gradually, symptoms begin to emerge:

- Blurry vision

- Distorted visual images

- Double vision

- Increasing nearsightedness

- Poor night vision

- Uncomfortable glare from sunlight or bright light

The treatments

- **Cataract surgery** is removing cataracts and replacing a substitute lens. However, a cataract surgery does not have to be performed immediately, nor is the procedure absolutely necessary, depending on the quality of the vision.

- **Eye drops** may be used to dilate the pupils to allow greater transmission of light to the retina.

- **Stronger lighting** may have to be employed for close work. Positioning lighting directly over reading material and using frosted light bulbs to reduce glare are some of the practical measures to improve poor vision due to cataracts.

- **Reading point by point** may help preventing cataracts from deteriorating. Seeing details is done through the **macula**, which is the center point of the retina. But the macula can see only a small portion of the visual field at a time. Therefore, constantly shifting the eye can enhance the macula, while straining to take in the entire visual field all at once can weaken the macula. Accordingly, reading point by point, although it may be slower, helps strengthening the macula, and hence instrumental in maintaining detailed vision.

Practice the **elephant swing exercise** (See CHAPTER FIVE.) to increase your detailed vision and make shifting automatic. When you shift your eyes automatically and constantly, you are efficiently using your macula.

FOUR

THE BATES METHOD

WHAT IS THE BATES METHOD?

The natural vision improvement in this book is based on the vision system of the world-famous **William Bates**, M.D.; as a matter of fact, all the natural vision improvement programs currently available are all based on his original vision theories with different modifications over the past century.

Dr. William Bates demonstrated a very revolutionary natural approach to vision and eye care.

Here is a simple explanation of his method, now known as **The Bates Method**.

Dr. Bates' Theories of Vision

The Bates Method is actually a very simple and natural way to correct vision. Because it is so natural and harmless, it has become more widely known and recognized after many decades of controversy and debates. Today, many scientists still find it difficult to accept some of his unconventional theories of vision.

Dr. Bates' fundamental theories are as follows:

- The conditions of the eye are constantly changing, resulting in constant changes in the shape of the eyeball.

- The focus of the eye is constantly changing too (it is always looking at close and distant objects), resulting in the constant shifting of the eye.

The human eye is able to see in spite of these constant changes in the eye because the normal eye can adapt or adjust to these changes—known as "**eye accommodation.**"

However, eye accommodation may deteriorate due to many factors, such as weak eye muscles, poor light conditions, impaired macula (responsible for visual details). After all, the eye is just another body organ, which, like other body organs, is also vulnerable to disease and degeneration. When that happens, the eye cannot accommodate itself to see clearly, resulting in blurry vision.

It is universally accepted that weak vision occurs when the light from a close or distant object falls not precisely on the retina of the human eye—instead, it falls *in front of* (**nearsightedness**) or *behind* the retina (**farsightedness**).

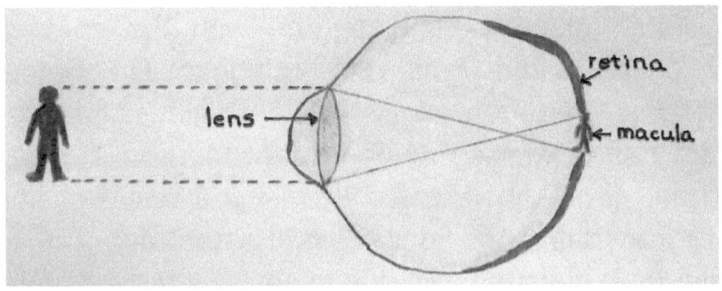

The Conventional Treatment of Weak Vision

To correct weak vision or **refractive error** (light not properly refracted on the retina of the eye), the conventional treatment by ophthalmologists and opticians is to make use of **corrective lenses** (eyeglasses or contacts) with proper prescriptions to enable the light from a close or distant object to refract accurately on the retina.

The conventional treatment serves two purposes:

- To make the eye see more clearly

- To prevent further eyestrain through clearer vision

These are the sole reasons for the professionals to provide eyeglasses and contacts: to provide better vision, and to prevent more eyestrain.

The conventional treatment is based on the belief that weak vision is due to incorrect refraction on the retina because of the distorted eye lens; therefore, to correct the impaired vision, corrective lenses are used to correct the refraction from the distorted lens.

Dr. Bates' Treatment of Weak Vision

Dr. Bates completely disagreed with the conventional theory of **distorted lens**. According to Dr. Bates, the conventional treatment is WRONG because the eye is constantly changing, so much so that the eye prescriptions (which are constant) in corrective lenses may not help the patients in certain conditions; quite the contrary, they unduly increase their eyestrain. That is to say, if the eye is forced to see in *different* eye conditions with the *same* corrective lenses, the eye will have to strain itself to see in different conditions, and thus causing further eyestrain that damages vision.

Dr. Bates' explanation was that what might fit the eye (i.e. the prescriptions) at one moment might not be appropriate at another moment, given that the conditions of the eye are constantly changing. In addition, because the eye is capable of *adapting* and *adjusting* to different conditions (eye accommodation), wearing corrective lenses will deprive the eye of such accommodation, and thus leading to further vision deterioration. *That* was the reason for his objection to wearing corrective lenses.

Dr. Bates' treatment was based on the belief that the incorrect refraction on the retina is due to weak and unrelaxed eye muscles, which cause **distorted shape in the eyeball**, resulting in the refraction falling in front of or behind the retina, instead of directly on the retina.

Nearsightedness: the lens becoming flattened

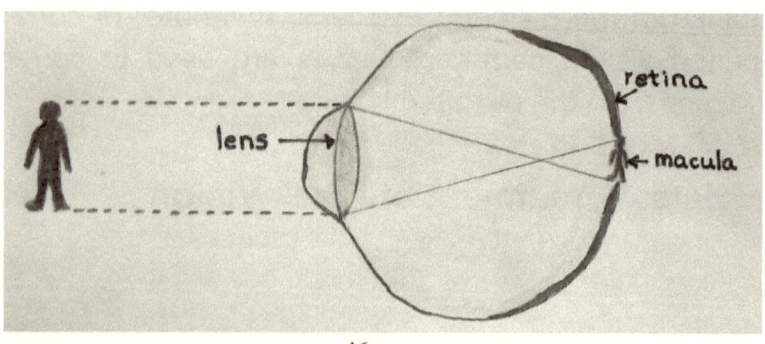

Farsightedness: the lens becoming thicker

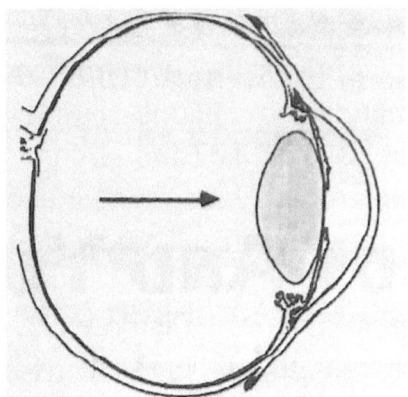

Accordingly, **eye relaxation** holds the key to correcting vision problems.

The normal eyeball is round. According to Dr. Bates, if you **strain** to see, your eyeball becomes distorted. As a result, you cannot see clearly. Because you cannot see, you strain your eyes more. The more you strain your eyes, the less you will be able to see, and thus forming a vicious circle of poor vision. The Bates Method is to break that vicious circle of eyestrain.

Unfortunately, you cannot *consciously* control your eye muscles. That is to say, you cannot tell your eye muscles not to squeeze your eyes out of shape. What you can do is to control them *unconsciously* through **awareness**, which is what this book is all about.

Below is a brief comparison between Dr. Bates' method and the conventional method of vision treatment:

Fact: Weak vision is due to **incorrect refraction**—either in front of or behind, but not directly *on* the retina.

Bates' Treatment Theory: Distorted shape of the eyeball, due to weak and un-relaxed eye muscles, causes the incorrect refraction on the eye's retina.

Solution: Strengthen and relax eye muscles to prevent them from squeezing the eye out of shape when focusing.

Recommendation: Corrective lenses only create the desire for clear vision but deprives the eye from *naturally* adjusting to the constant changing conditions of the eye, and thus causing eyestrain as a result. Stop wearing your corrective lenses. Instead, relax your eye muscles to improve your vision such that you can ultimately do without your glasses.

Conventional Treatment Theory: Distorted eye lens causes the incorrect refraction on the eye's retina.

Solution: Use corrective lens to re-adjust the refraction on the retina in order to give clearer vision and to prevent further eyestrain.

Recommendation: Just continue to wear your corrective lenses. If vision changes, get a new pair.

The Bates Method focuses on the following basic principles of good vision:

- **Central fixation**: Train the eye to focus on only *one point one at a time*. To illustrate, let your eyes look at a printed page:

    - Focus on only **one word** on the printed page, allowing other words in its vicinity to become blurred.

    - Then, try to see **one letter** of that word *better* than the other letters of that word.

    - Then, look at the **other letters**, one by one.

❖ Now, look at the **blank space** between that word and the next.

❖ Focus on the next word, and repeat the process.

The objective of this training is to help you focus on only a very small area because the **macula** (responsible for detailed vision) can see only a very small area. Stimulate the macula to enhance vision improvement.

- **Shifting**: Train the eye to look from one object to another frequently, from a close object to a distant one, and then back again in order to relieve tension and eyestrain, which impair good vision. Reinforce shifting with constant **blinking** to clean and to rest the eye. (See **blinking** in CHAPTER FIVE.)

- **Sunning**: Train the eye to adapt and adjust to bright light to avoid squinting, which causes eyestrain. Close your eyes and look up at the sun. Then, turn away from the sun, opening your eyes, and look at some clouds. Close your eyes for a moment, and then open your eyes at look at a point a little nearer the sun, but without looking directly at the sun. Sunning sharpens your vision, as well as prevents squinting. (See **sunning** in CHAPTER FIVE.)

- **Relaxation**: Visualizing "black" induces complete relaxation of the eye. A completely relaxed eye will see only black when it is closed; seeing the field of vision grayish or light-golden in color means that the eye is not *totally* relaxed. **Eye palming** is the most effective exercise for complete eye relaxation. (Go to <u>CHAPTER FIVE</u> to find out how to **use eye palming** to relax.)

FIVE

NATURAL VISION IMPROVEMENT

EYE VISION

What Is Vision?

Vision is all about light. Without light, there is no vision.

"In the beginning, when God created the universe, the earth was formless and desolate. The raging ocean that covered everything was engulfed in total darkness, and the power of God was moving over the water. Then God commanded, 'Let there be light'—and light appeared." (**Genesis** 1-3)

Give that vision is a gift from God, do not abuse it; make the best and the most of your vision power. Improve your vision at any age!

Vision is about *how* your eyes make use of light to see the world around you:

- How much light is available to the eye?

- How efficient is the eye lens in refracting the light?

- How sensitive is the eye (macula) in receiving and transmitting the light to the brain?

- How proficient is the brain in processing the visual data from the eye?

Vision involves more than just the eye: it includes the body and the mind.

- So, never strain the eye to read or to see when the light is insufficient.

- So, relax the eye in order to avoid distorting the shape of the eye, which will squeeze the lens out of shape, and thus causing the refractive error.

- So, protect the macula (for detailed vision) on the retina (the back of the eye) by increasing peripheral vision (on both sides) to avoid overusing the macula.

- So, improve brain power through affirmations and visualization to help the eye focus and process visual information efficiently.

Good Vision

Good vision means the capability to look clearly into the distance, but *nearsightedness* causes blurry distance.

Good vision means having peripheral vision, but the grim reality is that there is only central vision, with little or no periphery.

Good vision means the eyes shift constantly, but the problem is that the eyes are constantly staring, or have developed eye-fixation.

Good vision means the eyes can adjust easily to light, but the truth of the matter is that the eyes tend to squint at different light conditions.

Good vision means the eyes can look close up and far away almost instantaneously, but *farsightedness* prevents the instant shifting of the eyes.

In other words, the characteristics of the eye with good vision are:

- It will "**naturally observe**" or "**notice**" what is around.

- It will never "**strain**" to see "**everything**."

- It will **relax** and **rest** even when it is "**looking**."

To improve vision is to enhance and to maintain these characteristics *at all times*.

HOW DOES THE EYE "SEE"

The eye with good vision and the eye with weak vision do not "see" in the same way. Understanding *how* normal eyes "see" may help you make your eyes "see" in a totally *different* way.

Look at a simple illustration of the difference in the process of "seeing" by the eye with good vision and by the eye with weak vision. Here is *how* and *what* the healthy eye will "see" when it looks at the following:

A B C D E

- The eye with good vision will be able to "absorb" or "see" **A**, **B**, **C**, **D**, and **E** *all at the same time*, irrespective of the closeness or distance.

- Then, the eye with good vision will subconsciously "select" the one (e.g. **E**) that it wants to see, and immediately shifting its focus to **E**. Remember, the healthy eye can "select" its own vision.

In other words, the healthy eye has "**soft vision**"—it sees *everything immediately but without gazing.* "Soft vision" is practiced by all martial arts practitioners because they need to know *where* the attack of the enemy may be coming from—which could be from *any* or *all* directions. Therefore, it is important to train your eyes to have "soft vision" so that you can see *everything all at once.*

Soft Focus

Train your eyes to "see" and "look" *at the same time.*

- Look at a printed page with a lot of details.

- Become "aware" of what you are looking at, without blinking your eyes for five to thirty seconds.

Practice soft focus for five minutes at least once a day.

AWARENESS: Look without blinking (soft vision) for 10 seconds or so.

When you gaze, you use mostly your central vision, with little or no peripheral vision (which is side vision); accordingly, you weaken your macula, which is responsible for seeing visual details. Over time, you begin to lose much of your peripheral vision (use it or lose it). Because you cannot see what you want to see, you form the bad habit of "staring" or "frozen gaze," and thus further weakening your macula. This is how the vicious circle of poor vision is formed. To improve your vision, you must break that vicious circle.

The eye with weak vision will do the following when looking at the above:

- The eye with weak vision will probably look *consciously* at C *first*, without seeing the other alphabets (probably due to constant use of central vision).

- Then, the eye with weak vision may probably shift its gaze to B and D, and then to A and E, back and forth, in order to "select" what it wants to see. Finally, the eye may decide that E is what it wants to see, and begins to focus on E (all these happen subconsciously and within only a fraction of a split second).

The above illustration demonstrates *how* the eye with weak vision may "see." One of the characteristics of the eye with weak vision is its "frozen gaze," which allows it to focus on only *one object one at a time*. To improve your vision, you must overcome the bad habit of "staring."

AWARENESS: Do not stare!. Blink frequently to stop frozen gaze!

VISION IMPROVEMENT

Vision improvement is based on the **four principles** of good vision:

- Relaxing the eye

- Strengthening the eye

- Adjusting the eye to light

- Balancing the eye

Relaxing the Eye

Eye relaxation begins with the mind *first*, not the eye. The mind must be *completely* relaxed before it can relax the body—and the eye, which is only one of the many organs of the body.

Practice **meditation** daily. (See CHAPTER TWO.)

Relax the body to relax the eye

Practicing Oriental exercises, such as **Qi Gong**, **Tai Chi**, and **Yoga**, can significantly relax the body because these exercises focus on "soft" movements of the body. Western-style exercises, on the other hand, focus more on building physical strength and muscles rather than on relaxing the muscles.

Do some, if not all, of the following exercises to relax the body, and hence prepare you for exercises to relax the eye.

The neck

- Stand with your feet slightly apart, and knees at ease.

- Firm your lower abdominal muscles, and straighten your upper back.

- Loosen your shoulders, and let them face forward.

- Let your head fall backward for a count of 10

- Slowly turn your head to the left and then to the right, each for a count of 5.

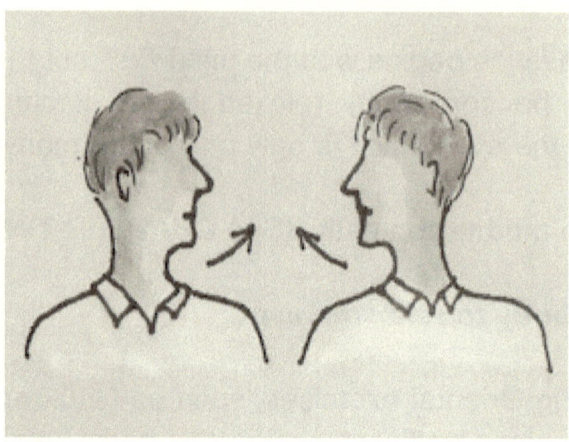

- With shoulders facing forward, move your head to look up and down, each for a count of 5.

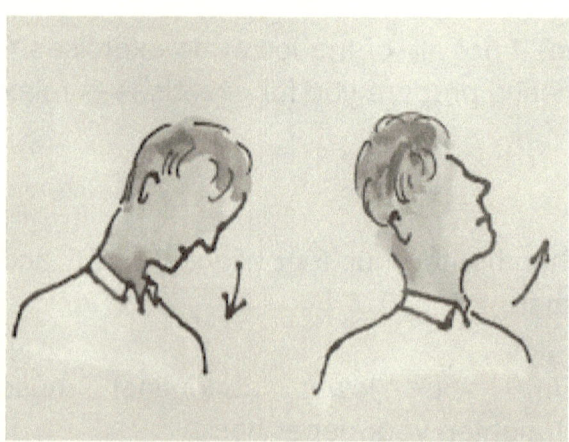

- With shoulders facing forward, move your head sideways, bringing the left ear to the left shoulder, and then the right ear to the right shoulder, each for a count of 5.

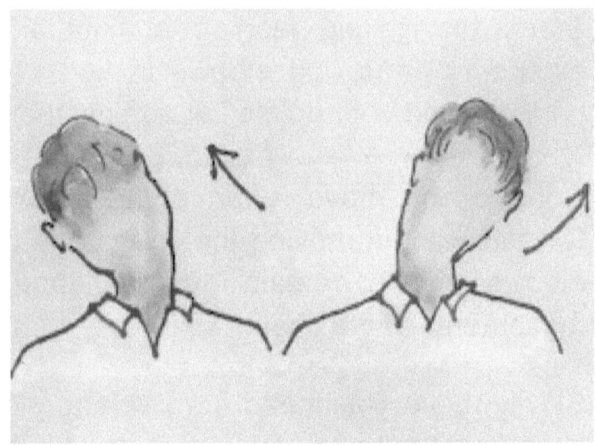

- Repeat the above.

The neck exercises can be practiced at any time—even when you are at work or waiting for the bus. Always keep your neck muscles relaxed and supple.

The upper torso

- Interlace your fingers of both hands, with palms towards you.

- Slowly move your arms in a large circle, reaching as far as you can without straining your arm and shoulder muscles.

- Repeat a few circles in a clockwise direction, and then in an anti-clockwise direction.

The chest, neck, and head

- Stand facing and leaning against a wall, with extending arms and elbows locked in a straight position, and your palms flat against the wall.

- Consciously move your chest backward and forward without moving the rest of the body. Your elbows should remain straight throughout the movements of the chest.

- Slowly move your head from side to side as your chest puffs out and caves in during your inhalation and exhalation.

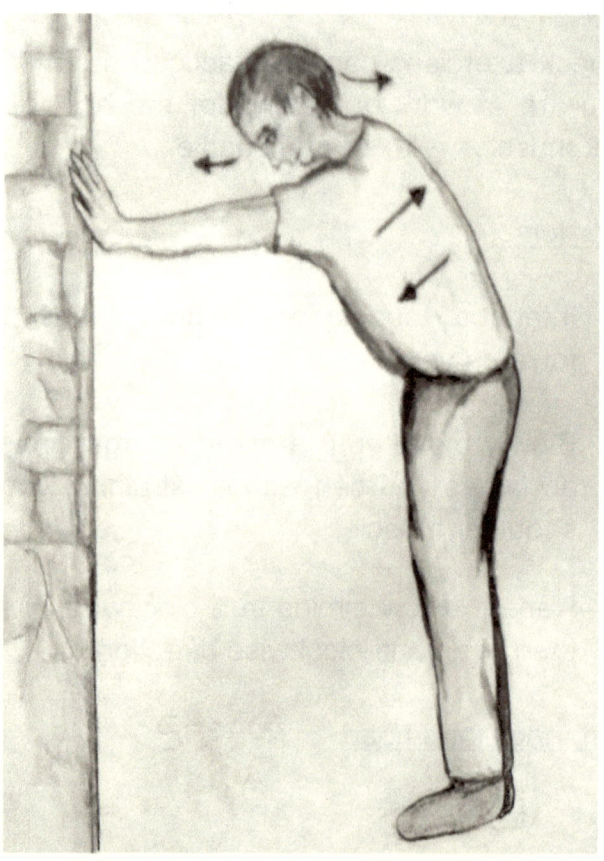

Stretching and Curling

- Stand with your feet close together.

- Inhale deeply and stretch up, and then from side to side. Give yourself a big yawn.

- Take a deep breath. Exhale slowly as you relax your head forward and down, right and left. Open your eyes and "notice" the world around you.

- Stretch up your hands above your head as far as you can go. Feel the stretch on your sides. Breathe slowly, and count 10.

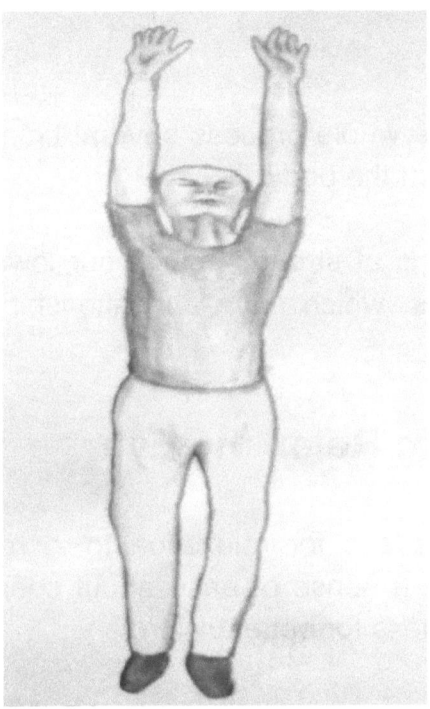

- Keeping your knees a little bent, curl your body forward until your hands touch the floor. Keep your neck, hands and shoulders relaxed. Look upward with your eyes to keep your spine straight. Remain in this position for a count of 10.

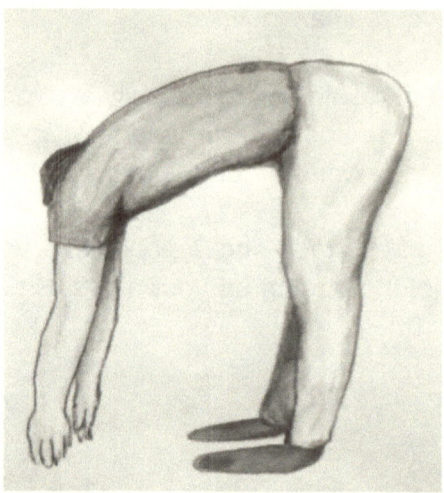

- Repeat the whole process several times for deep relaxation of the body.

This exercise aims at strengthening your lower back as well as your kidneys, which have a relationship with your eyes.

Self-Massage to Relax the Eye

Self-massage the eye for relaxation to increase blood circulation, to create a sense of ease about seeing, and to enhance eye awareness for better vision.

Facial and eye massage

- Breathe deeply and slowly.

- Rub both hands to generate warmth.

- Massage your **jaw** with your hands moving in small circles, from the chin outward along your jawbone up to the front of and behind your ears.

- Then, move your hands over the bridge of your nose, and massage outward along your **cheekbones** until you reach your temples and your ears.

- Then, starting from the bridge of your nose, massage along your **eyebrows**, moving above, below, and along the brow. Use your thumbs to press against the grooves slightly below your eyebrow ridge close to the bridge of your nose.

- Gently squeeze your **eyeball** with your fingers.

- Finally, use long, firm, strokes to massage your **forehead** from the left to the right, and then the right to the left.

Throughout your facial and eye self-massage, look for **sore spots**, especially in the eyebrow area. Massage them with slightly harder and stronger circular movements.

Rubbing the eye

- Apply and press the heel of your left palm and the heel of your right palm against your left eye and right eye, respectively.

- With gentle pressure, rub with a twisting movement your left eye with your left palm and your right eye with your right palm.

- Meanwhile, contract and relax your eyelid muscles.

Acupressure for eye massage and eye relaxation

Apply pressure and massage from your fingers to stimulate all the acupressure/acupuncture points around your eyes.

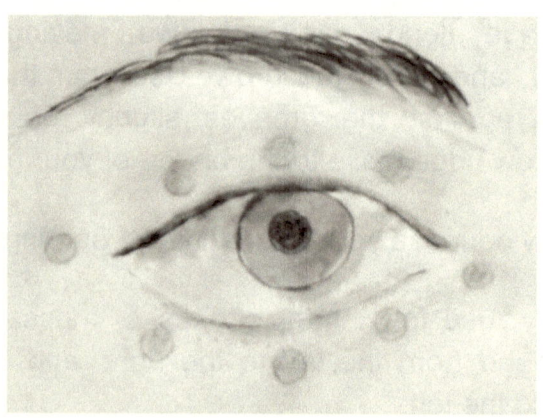

The hoku point: Applying pressure to the hoku points of your hands can effectively relieve headaches because the hoku points control the organs of the head and the eyes.

- Place the *thumb* of your right hand on the **muscular hill** of your left hand, with the index finger of the right hand on the inside of the left hand corresponding to the point of the muscular hill.

- Apply pressure of the right thumb and the right index finger against each other, while breathing naturally in and out.
- Repeat this using the left thumb and the left index finger on the right hand.

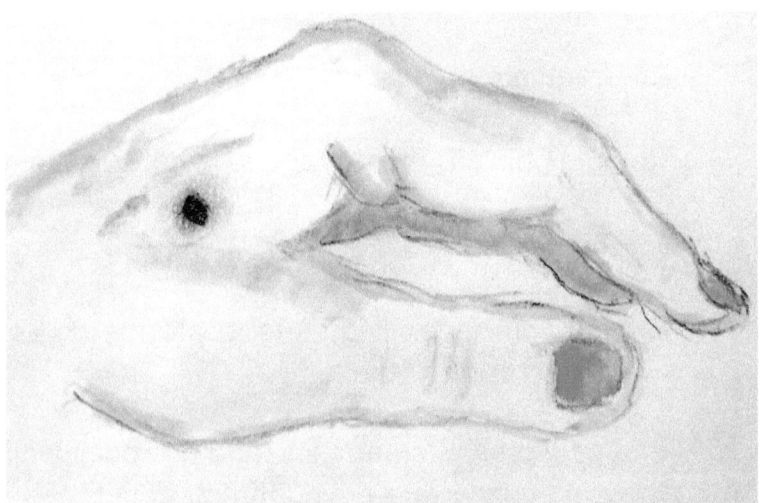

Press the "muscular hill" both on the outside and the inside.

The eyebrow point: This massage relaxes the eye and promotes better blood circulation to the eye.

- Gently close your eyes.

- Use your thumbs to apply pressure to or massage the inside corners of your eyebrows to relieve eye pressure due to eyestrain.

- Breathe naturally.

The nose point: This massage improves breathing and relaxes the eye.

- Gently close your eyes.

- Use your thumb and index finger over the bridge of your nose to massage the nose point for eye relaxation.

- Breathe naturally.

The temple point: This massage relieves eyestrain.

- Gently close your eyes.

- Use your index fingers to locate the hollow space on each side of the temple.

- Apply pressure and massage this point while being fully aware of your breaths.

The eyebrow-and-cheek points: This massage not only relieves tightness due to eyestrain but also promotes better breathing.

- Gently close your eyes.

- Use your index and middle fingers of each hand to massage all your eyebrow-and-cheek points simultaneously.

- Be aware of your breaths.

The occipital points: The occipital points are located between your ears in the back lower part of your head—the meeting points of the muscles of spine up at the back of your neck. Stimulating these acupressure points relaxes not only the neck but also the eye, which has a close connection with the neck and the head.

- Apply deep pressure with the sides of your thumbs, or your fingertips for 1 to 2 minutes.

- Meanwhile, look straight ahead, and breathe naturally.

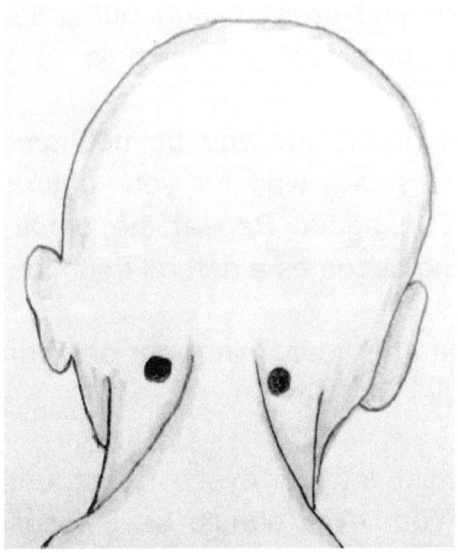

The occipital points behind the neck

Regular Eye Relaxation

To overcome eyestrain, which causes weak eye muscles, you need regular eye relaxation for optimum vision health:

- Consciously breathe in and breathe out through your nose to bring more oxygen to your eyes, as well as to reduce any stress on your vision. (Learn **diaphragm breathing** and **alternate-nostril breathing** from CHAPTER TWO.)

- Loosen your shoulders and keep them down to allow as much oxygen as possible to fill up your lungs as you breathe in through your nose.

- Push out as much as possible the carbon dioxide from the bottom of your lungs, feeling your stomach and chest flatten out gradually as you breathe out through your nostrils.

  It is important that you do not *force* yourself to *inhale*; instead, wait for your natural impulse to breathe in again. Repeat the process until your breathing becomes a natural rhythm.

  Concentrate your mind on only breathing and nothing else.

- Meanwhile, let your eyelids droop until they gently close. Your eyes should be *unfocused* and your eye muscles *relaxed*. Slightly open your mouth, while dropping your jaw.

- Continue breathing for a few minutes with your eyes closed.

- Now, open your eyes. When you re-open your eyes, do not focus immediately on anything in particular.

- Blink your eyes repeatedly to soothe and moisturize your eyes. If possible, induce self-yawning.

- Smile broadly and hold for five seconds to remove any tension you might be holding in your eyes.

Practice eye relaxation as often as required, especially when you feel eyestrain, for vision health.

Eye palming to relax the Eye

This unique eye-relaxation exercise uses your healing hands to direct energy to your eyes, as well as to rest your optic nerve and relax your entire nervous system.

Unlike sleep, which is unconscious and passive relaxation, palming is conscious and active relaxation. Therefore, palming is one of the best exercises for eye relaxation. Practice palming at least for 10 to 30 minutes per session for three or more sessions daily to completely relax your eyes. Even at work, you can palm your eyes for 2 minutes, if possible, to relieve your eyestrain from the computer.

- Sit comfortably with your elbows resting on a table in front of you—preferably in a darkened room, such as a bathroom without any window.

- Rub your palms together to generate some warmth.

- Place your palms over your eyes, without touching them, while resting them on the boney ridge surrounding your eyes with the heels of your hands on your cheekbones. Your eyes should be *gently* closed.

- Relax your mind, and breathe deeply through your nose, not your mouth. The slower your breathing is, the more relaxed your mind becomes.

- Feel your abdomen and back expand and contract as you inhale and exhale, respectively.

- Visualize complete darkness to relax your mind.

- Feel your neck and shoulders expand and contract as your deep and slow breathing continues.

- Visualize every part of your body—hands, fingers, toes, knees, and thighs—expand and contract with your inhalation and exhalation.

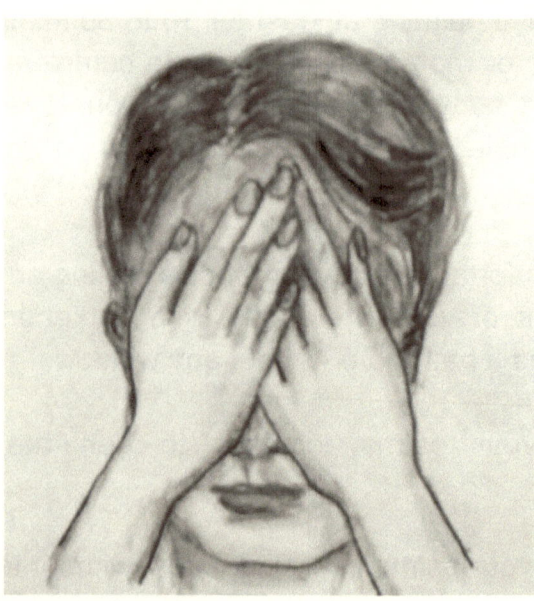

Practice eye palming whenever you feel fatigue in your

eyes. It is impossible to palm for too long or for too much; some palm for hours to reap the benefits of both relaxation and meditation. If you feel any resistance to palming, it may probably be due to your subconscious resistance to relaxation. If you become more relaxed, you will see complete blackness. However, it is all right if you do not see complete blackness; just continue with your daily palming exercise.

Remember, we are living in a stressful world, and many of us simply cannot relax, even if we very much would like to. Attesting to the inability to relax, many of us easily and often stare without blinking—and, worse, without being aware of it. As a result, our vision slowly and gradually deteriorates over the years.

Do not let a day pass by without palming your eyes.

The "8" eye exercise

Do the following "8" eye exercise as often as required to relax your eye muscles as well to increase their flexibility.

- Sit comfortably in a relaxed posture.

- Consciously breathe in and breathe out through your nose until you attain a natural rhythm.

- Imagine the figure "8" in the distance.

- Let your eyes *trace* along the imaginary figure without moving your head.

- First, trace it in one direction, and then in the opposite direction.

You can modify the exercise by imagining other alphabets and figures. The objective of this exercise, in addition to promoting relaxation and flexibility, is to train your eyes to consciously shift when focusing on an object in the distance.

The Taoist squeeze-and-open eye exercise

This ancient Chinese exercise developed by Taoist monks thousands of years ago increases blood circulation to the eyes, prevents watery eyes, and alkalizes the eyes to detoxify the liver. It removes eyestrain and soothes eye-muscle tension.

- Inhale slowly, while squeezing your eyes *tightly* for 10 seconds.

- Then, slowly exhale your breath, making the sh-h-h-h-h sound, while opening your eyes wide.

- Repeat as many times and as often as required to cleanse the eyes and the liver.

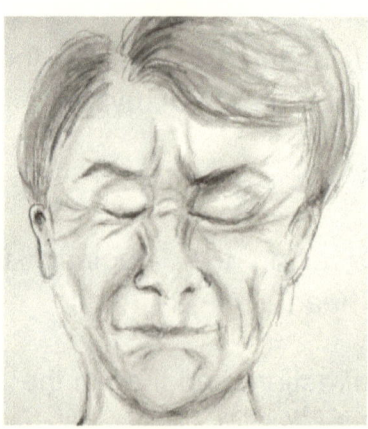 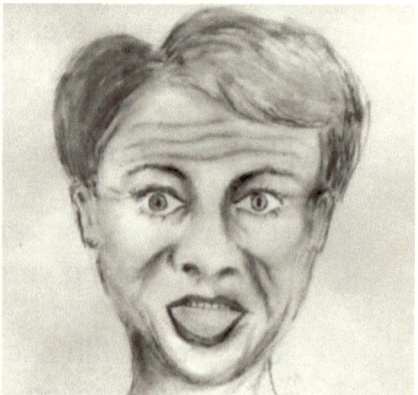

Squeeze and open to relax.

The Chinese "yang" eye candle gazing

Practice this ancient Chinese eyesight-improvement technique to clear the whites of the eye in order to sharpen vision and to relax the eye through cleansing.

- Sit comfortably.

- Light a candle and place it at arm's length and at eye level in front of you.

- Gaze at the flame without blinking your eyes.

- Allow tears to flow out from your eyes (they remove toxins from your body).

- If need be, close your eyes for 10 seconds every now and then.

Practice it daily for at least 5 minutes. End your gazing session by closing your eyes and do the **palming exercise** for a few minutes to cool down your eyes.

Stretching eye muscles for relaxation

Master the eye-muscle stretching exercise to relieve eye tension and maintain relaxation.

- Sit comfortably, taking a few deep breaths.

- Stretch your eyes upward as far as they can go without straining them.

- Hold your breath. Stretch your eyes downward as you exhale.

- Repeat this up and down movements of your eyes a few times.

- Stretch your eyes by moving them around in circles, but without straining them, as you breathe in and breathe out.

Perform this exercise anytime and anywhere, such as waiting for the bus, standing in line, or walking.

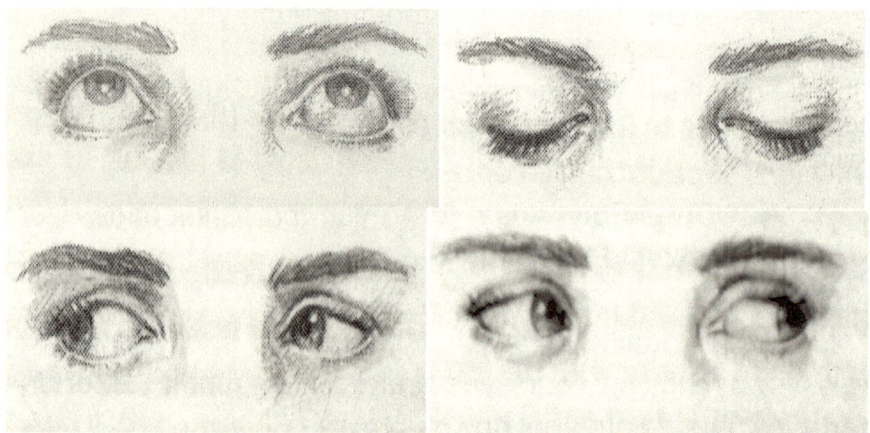

Yawning to cleanse and relax the eye

Yawning is a natural way to relax the body and the mind, as well as to cleanse the eye.

- Practice yawning deliberately with wide-open jaws, while expelling sounds through your mouth. If possible, induce tears from your eyes.

- After a few yawns, close your eyes, and relax.

- Now, with eyes closed, use your nose to draw the figure "8" vertically, horizontally, and diagonally (nose painting).

With practice, you can yawn anytime and anywhere, even when you are not tired.

Strengthening the Eye

If you overuse your muscles, you stress and strain them; if you under use them, you may develop muscle atrophy. In the same manner, you must improve your vision through both **rest** and **use**. That is to say, you relax and strengthen your eyes to improve your vision.

Learn how to blink

If you do not blink frequently enough, you will not be able to see well. It is just that simple. Blinking has many vision benefits:

- It overcomes the harmful habit of staring.

- It relaxes the eye.

- It cleanses and massages the eye.

- It improves nearsightedness.

Learn how to blink, not squint. The former relaxes the eye, while the latter stresses the eye because it uses undue force to close and open the eye.

Practice the following to make blinking second nature to you:

- Breathe deeply.

- Close and open your eyes. The blink has to be soft, not hard, and it must be complete. Imagine using your eyelashes to cause your eyes to close and open. Practice this several times until you master it. You may even count while you blink to make sure you do not blink too fast.

- Close your right eye, and cover it with your right hand.

- Blink your left eye. If the blink is soft, and not forced, your right hand over your right eye will not feel any movement. It is important that your blinking has to be soft and effortless.

- Repeat the process with the other eye.

Always remember to blink several times before you look at something in close vision and in distant vision. Habit forming is important.

AWARENESS: Always blink—soft and complete! Form the habit of constant blinking.

Learn how to increase peripheral vision

The macula in the center of the retina is responsible for detailed vision. Overuse of the central vision leads to weakening of the macula, resulting in much loss of detailed vision.

Increasing peripheral vision will decrease the use of central vision, and hence instrumental in protecting the macula and enhancing detailed vision, which is critical to good vision.

- Cut small black rectangular cards in different sizes (2"x 2"; 2"x3"; 2"x5") from construction paper. Tape the card to the top of the bridge of your nose, covering part of both eyes.

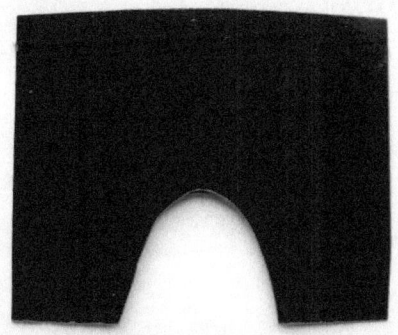

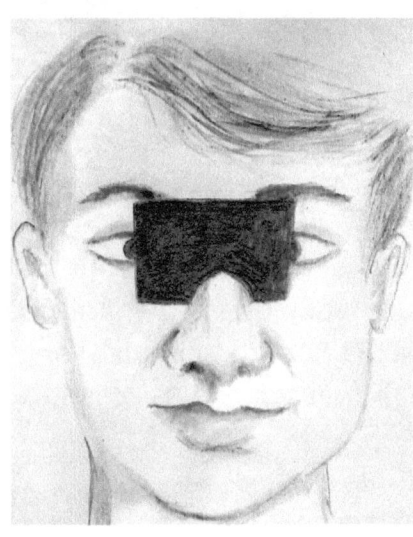

- Sit or stand, and look through the smallest black rectangular card in front of your eyes, while turning your head from side to side.

- Notice that your surrounding seems to be "moving" in the opposite direction.
- Stop turning your head, and close your eyes for a minute or two. Now, visualize the previous "moving surrounding" in your mind's eye.

- Open your eyes again, and move or wave your hands on both sides of your ears. Notice your moving hands, which are now stimulating your peripheral cells.

- Stop waving your hands, and close your eyes. Now, visualize the movement of your hands in your mind's eye.

- Repeat the above with the mid-size and then the large-size black rectangular cards.

By partially covering the eyes, your mind enables your eyes to pay more attention to what is on both sides, and hence stimulates your peripheral vision. After each exercise, you will see that your vision has "expanded" and has become "broad." By strengthening your peripheral vision, you indirectly reduce your use of central vision, and hence protecting your macula from deterioration and degeneration.

AWARENESS: Ttrain your eyes to see what is on both sides of your eyes.

Learn how to shift and swing

The elephant swing

Practice this basic Qi Gong exercise—the elephant swing—to enhance circulation, relaxation, peripheral vision, soft vision, and integration of vision. This is an excellent exercise for overall vision improvement.

- Stand with your feet parallel, about 10 inches apart.

- Gently close your eyes.

- Shake your arms and legs, and roll your neck sideways, back and forth until they become soft and relaxed.

- Still your mind, and breathe naturally.

- Now, open your eyes, and look at what is in front of you.

- Slowly swing your body to the right and then to the left by shifting your weight from one foot to the other and lifting the heel of each foot as you turn in a swaying motion. Let your arms hang loosely, and let your head move with your body, not by itself.

- The surrounding seems to "move" in the opposite direction. Let your eyes "shift" naturally without fixing on anything.

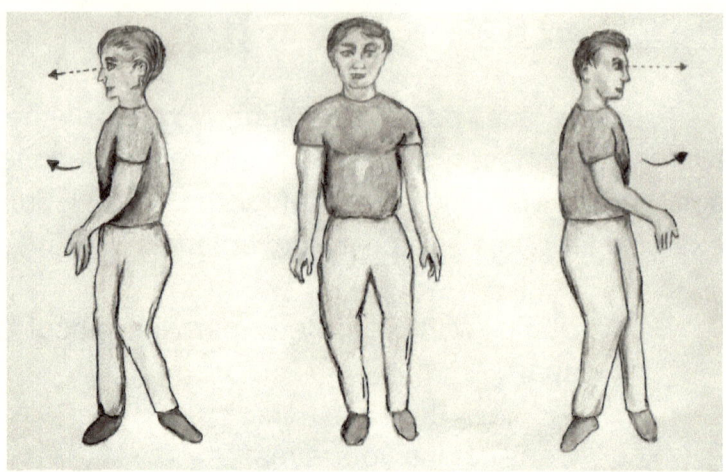

Another version of this exercise is to move your whole torso with your head, while your eyes are focusing on a finger held approximately 10 inches in front of your nose. Focusing on your thumb while swinging is an excellent way to train your eyes to see objects against a background.

Shifting

Shifting is natural and automatic movement of the eye. The normal eye makes several small movements every second. Natural shifting makes the eye look alert and alive.

Unfortunately, some cultures think that shifting the eye too often and too much may be an indication of dishonesty of character. As a result, some people may consciously begin to shift their eyes less, leading to staring or frozen gaze.

You see with the macula (the center of the retina) for sharp, detailed vision. If you see with other part of the eye, other than the macula, you will lose some of the details of your vision. Over time, your macula weakens, and your vision becomes less detailed, that is, you see only small portions of your visual field at any one time.

In addition to enhancing your periphery to strengthen

your macula by doing the **peripheral vision exercise** and the **elephant swing exercise** above, observe the following:

- Develop a "soft vision"—that is, seeing without straining.

- Stop wearing your eyeglasses or contacts as much as possible. Of course, you need them when you drive or do certain tasks that require clear vision, but there are times you do not need them, especially when you relax or are at home.

- Develop the mentality that you do not need to see everything in detail; wearing eyeglasses or contacts has conditioned your eyes to crave clarity in vision. So, if you don't see anything in clarity, you subconsciously strain your eyes in an attempt to "see better" and thus form the vicious circle of eyestrain and vision deterioration. This is how your eyesight has gone from bad to worse. To stop this vicious circle, give up the need to see better until you have improved your vision, and only when that happens then you will be able to see better. In short, a *temporary* blurry vision is OK.

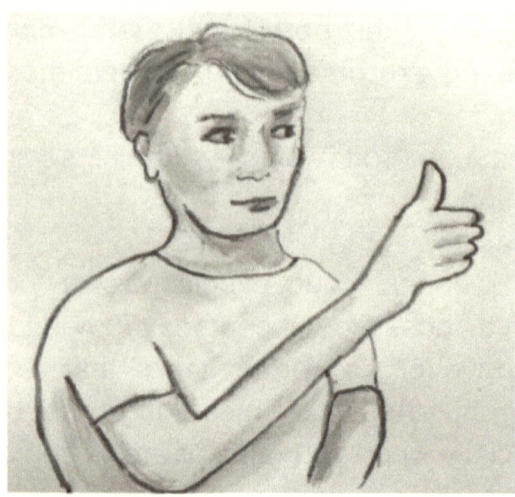

AWARENESS: Swing and shift for clear and soft vision!

Shifting is moving the eye from point to point. Shifting is seeing consciously without straining the eye. Train your eyes to look at distant objects by moving slowly around them, seeing the edge of each object.

Edging and Tracking

According to **Dr. William Bates**, the founder of natural vision, staring or fixation is the leading cause of loss of close and distant vision. To overcome this problem, practice **edging** and **tracking** as often as you can. Simply, develop this good vision habit.

- Edge and track letters on a printed page. Pick out smaller and smaller letters until you can read the smallest print easily.

- Edge and track distant objects to improve distant vision.

Edging or tracking can be done with your eyes only, or with your nose as a focal point (nose painting). Form the habit of edging and tracking while walking, looking out the window, reading, and so on. Every now and then, close your eyes to rest them. Practice edging or tracking (without glasses or contacts) as frequently as possible.

By the same token, you can also improve close vision by edging or tracking letters on a printed page by going around the outside and inside of the letter in print. Close your eyes every now and then. Practice this not only to improve close vision but also to relax the eye.

AWARENESS: Edge and track anytime and anywhere!

Corner shifting

Develop your **central fixation**, which is the ability of your eye to see one point best. It is not solely about the center of your sight; it is also the ability to see that for every single point of vision there are other details that may need to be observed too, right to the far edge of your periphery.

For example, look at the rectangle below. Shift your eyes from one corner to another corner, diagonally, back and forth, to promote relaxation and smooth eye movement. Most importantly, the exercise develops the awareness of central fixation.

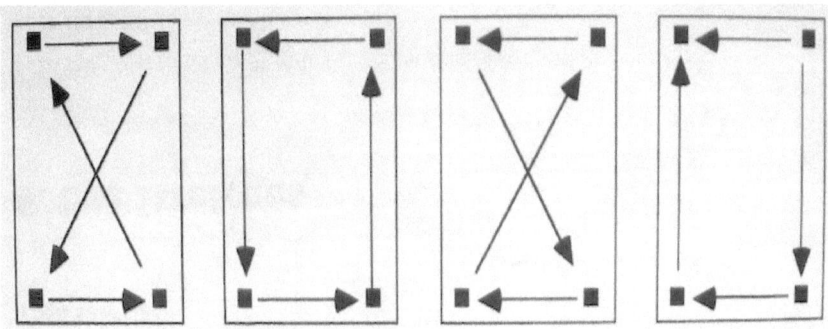

Finger shifting

- Hold up your two index fingers in front of your eyes, one at a distance of about 12 inches, and the other at arm's length.

- Look right through your near finger to the distant one. You have the optical illusion of seeing the first finger splitting into two.

- Now, shift your focus on the near finger close to your face.

- Keep your gaze on the near finger. Now, you have the optical illusion of seeing the other finger (the one at arm's length) splitting into two in the background.

- Shift back and forth; make sure you always see the other finger as two images

The objective of the finger shifting exercise is for visual adjustment to effectively coordinate your right eye and your left eye.

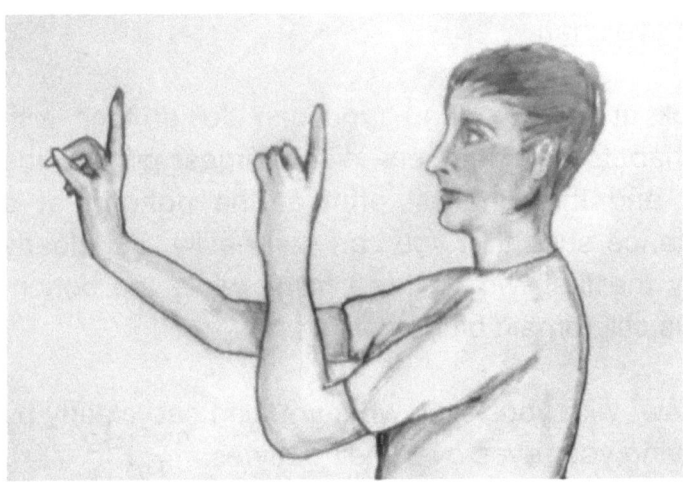

Looking at a picture

- Hold a picture with a lot of details in front of you—close enough that you can see some but not all of the details.

- Breathe naturally and be conscious of your breath.

- Find an object that you can see clearly. Use your eyes to edge or outline that object, shifting from one detail to another. For example, if you are looking at the picture of a house, use your eyes to trace its outline, and then shift to its windows, and the door, and the chimney, edging them one by one.

- Close your eyes, and visualize in your mind's eye the details that you have just observed.

- Now look at other details that might be blurry to you, and repeat the process.

Looking at an eye chart

- Look at an eye chart (you can design one with alphabets and numbers in the largest print at the top and the smallest print at the bottom) at a distance such that you can see easily and clearly only the first two or three rows, while the bottom rows still remain blurry.

- "Draw" with your eyes what you can see clearly by moving your eyes over their outlines.

- Simultaneously, wave your hands over your ears (just like what you do in the **peripheral vision training exercise**) to stimulate your peripheral vision.

- Gently close your eyes, and visualize in your mind's eye what you have just seen.

- Now, move to the next row below, line by line, and do the same.

- When you come to the line or row in which the alphabets and numbers look blurry to you, accept the blur. Remember, do not strain to see them. Do the same: shifting from one blur to another, and noticing the spaces between them.

When you finish a line, rest your eyes by going back to the original line and test how much your vision has improved.

Learn how to strengthen the eye accommodation

Your accommodative eye muscles weaken and deteriorate with age due to lack of use. Follow the ancient Hindu yogis eyesight-improving technique to strengthen your accommodative eye muscles so that you can see in the distance and also at close point. Most importantly, they enable your eyes to easily change focus through improving the eye muscles' flexibility.

- Write a few big black letters on a 2" x 3" card. Hold it at eye level and at arm's length away. Make sure you can see the letters clearly.

- Then, look at a distant object and see it clearly.

- Begin, one eye at a time, looking at the black letters at close distance and then looking at a distant object, and then with both eyes.

- Alternately, look at a close point object and a distant vision object.

- As your vision improves, move the card closer to you.

Zooming exercise is a variation of eye accommodation training: it is rapidly shifting your eye focus from a near distance to a far distance, back and forth.

- Sit comfortably with a one-eyed patch covering one eye, and your thumb in front of your other eye.

- Take a slow, deep breath.

- "Look" at your thumb in front of your eye (the distance from your eye should be such that the outline of your thumb remains clear and distinct), while "seeing" what is beyond your thumb. The more you are aware of the blur beyond your thumb, the clearer you will see your thumb.

- Now, "look" or focus on a distant object beyond your thumb. Try to edge or trace it, and then quickly shift back the focus on your thumb.

- Repeat the above back and forth.

- Practice zooming with the other eye.

The objective of zooming is to train and promote flexibility of focus between your mind and your eyes. Practice this exercise at least two to three times a day.

Learn how to focus

Practice the **ancient Egyptian black dot technique** to reshape your distorted eyeball by making the eye muscles focus in positions in which they do not normally focus.

- Draw a black dot (approximately ½ inch in diameter) on a white card (2" x 3").

- Hold the card at arm's length in front of you.

- Slowly move the card to the tip of your nose. Do not move your head. You should see only one dot; if you see two circles instead of one, move the card away from your nose until you can see the dot distinctly.

- Gaze at the black dot for 30 seconds. Then, close your eyes and rest for a few seconds.

- Next, raise the card between your eyebrows, move it as close as you can (make sure you can see clearly the dot), and gaze at the dot for another 30 seconds.

Learn how to stretch vision

- Stand straight in front of the **Snellen eye chart**. Look at one of the letters that you can see clearly.

- Mentally trace the letter with eyes closed. Relax the whole body, including your eyes.

- Open your eyes and look at the letter again.

- Place palms over your eyes, while visualizing the letter mentally for a few seconds.

- Open your eyes with a deep breath, and look at the letter yet again.

- Move back a little, and repeat the above sequence.

The objective of the stretch-vision exercise is to stretch your vision by enhancing vision through relaxation while increasing the distance from the object.

Learn how to see whole field of vision all at once

Looking at concentric circles makes you become more aware of how you are distorting part of the image.

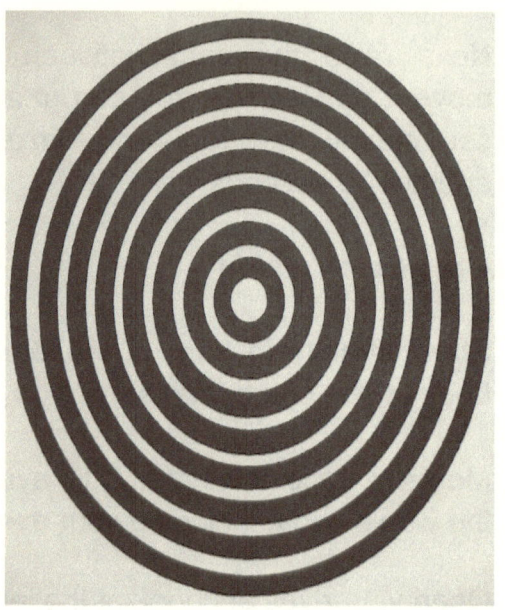

- Stand where you can see the center clearly. Notice how they continue all around the center.

- Move away from the concentric circles until they begin to "break."

- Now, relax your eyes through eye palming, blinking, and any other eye relaxation exercise until you can see the center in focus again.

- Repeat this back and forth.

Look at another picture:

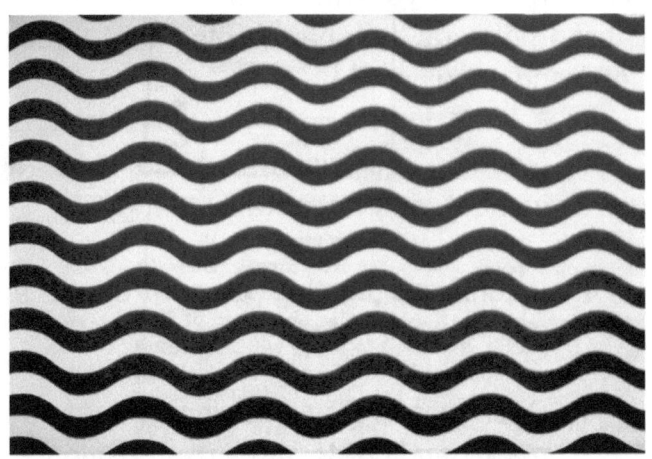

- Stand where you can see the black and white lines with the same width and running continuously.

- Move away until the black and white lines seem to have "broken."

- Now, relax your eyes through eye palming, blinking, and any other eye relaxation exercise until you can see the black and white lines in clear focus again, that is, running continuously.

The above optical illusion exercises train visual acuity and enhances near-point vision.

Learn how to read correctly

Biologically, you eyes are designed to adjust from close to distant focus, back and forth, *continually*. But, in reality, you focus your eyes for a long span of time at close distance when you read. This is one of the main causes of nearsightedness.

Reading causes **eyestrain**, which results in the

constriction of eye muscles. Prolonged eye muscle constriction distorts the shape of the eye. Eyestrain is due to the following conditions:

- Reading material being too close (less than 20 inches), and not parallel to the eye

- Insufficient lighting or too bright artificial lights (fluorescent lights)

- Poor posture in reading, such as slumping or neck-bending-downward position, leading to lengthening of the eyeball

- Reading while eating: digestion drawing blood to the digestive system, thereby temporarily depriving the eye of nutrients

To overcome eyestrain during reading, do the following:

- Breathe naturally; do not hold your breath.
- Take a meaningful break every 20 minutes or so, and blink your eyes repeatedly.

- Make sure the lighting is sufficient. Inadequate light is the first factor that tires the eye.

- Make sure the print is large enough.

It should be pointed out that **speed reading** may be damaging to the eye, because in speed reading the eye tends to take in a large visual field without focusing on any specific word. Remember, the macula can see small details only one at a time, that is, moving from one point to another.

If the macula cannot focus, it does *less* work, leading to more blurry vision, which ultimately increases eyestrain—and thus a vicious circle of eyestrain and weak vision.

To enhance vision in reading, do the following to focus on the physical aspect of reading:

- Occasionally read a page upside down, one letter at a time, moving from one point to another.

- Increase your peripheral vision and stimulate your macula by wearing black cardboard paper to partially cover the eyes.

Adjusting the Eye to Light

Given that light is the essence of good vision, it is therefore important that you train your eyes to adjust comfortably to light, otherwise you may have a tendency to squint your eyes when the light is too bright or too dim.

Eye sunning

Sunning the eye is an exercise that utilizes the energy from the sun for healing the eye and improving vision. The healing power of sunlight should come into the eye at a diagonal angle, and the sunlight should not be too strong (i.e. early in the morning, before 10 a.m. and late in the evening, after 5 p.m.)

- Sit or stand outdoors, your body facing the sun. You can also sit or stand at an open window, but do not let the sun come through glass.

- Close your eyes; do not wear sunglasses. Let the warm sunlight bathe your eyes.

- Now, move your head slowly but constantly from side to side.

- Breathe deeply and slowly.

- Relax your head, shoulders, and eyes, while continuing the body motion.

- Turn your back to the sun, and briefly palm your eyes for a few minutes during which you visualize black in your mind's eye.

- Return to the original position, and resume your eye sunning.

- Alternate between sunning and palming. You will notice that during sunning, the color seems brighter, while the black seems blacker during palming.

- Practice this for 10 to 20 minutes a day, if the weather permits.

Sun flashing

Flashing stimulates **retinal activity**

- Sit or stand with closed eyes facing the sun.

- Spread your fingers apart, and wave your hands back and forth across each other in front of your closed yes.

- Wave your hands more rapidly up and down past each other. You will see the interplay of darkness and light.

- Do palming for a few minutes, while visualizing black.

- Blink your closed eyes before you open them so they can readjust to light.

It is important that you never look directly into the sun, and that you do not practice sunning when the sunlight is too strong so as not to damage the eye.

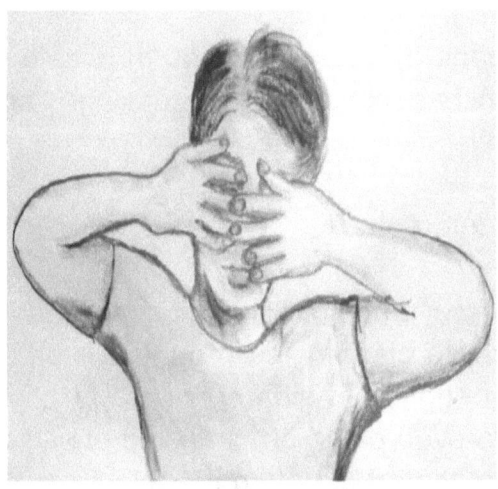

Flashing in the sun

The objective of eye sunning is to relax the eye and to help it adjust easily to light so as to avoid squinting during transition from darkness to light or from light to darkness.

Balancing the Eye

Wearing one-eyed patch

Wearing one-eyed patch (obtainable at your local pharmacy; or simply cover one of the lenses of your eyeglasses with a piece of paper) over an extended period of time (starting with half an hour, and extending to two to three hours a day) can stimulate and enhance your visual perceptions such that you will see *equally well* out of *both* eyes.

- Cover your "preferred eye" (the eye you would normally use if you were looking through, say, a telescope) with the eye patch.

- Engage in doing activities in a safe environment, such as cooking, exercising, and watching television at home.

Wearing two-eyed patch

Wearing two-eyed patch enhances your *peripheral vision*, which is critical to clearer and broader vision; it trains your awareness of peripheral vision.

Make a two-eyed patch out of a strip of stiff cardboard (3" x 1"), with a small part cut off in the middle to accommodate your nose. If you are wearing glasses, use adhesive tape to attach it to your eyeglasses. However, it is important that you should try to use your eye-patches *without* your glasses.

SIX

VISION NUTRITION

The prerequisite for vision health is vision nutrition, which builds healthy eye muscles, nerves, and blood vessels—the components of healthy eyes and perfect vision.

Self-healing is your own personal responsibility, just as **Hippocrates**, the father of medicine, once said: "Your food should be your medicine, and your medicine should be your food." Make food your medicine. Heal your eye problems and improve your vision with diet and nutrition. Vision nutrition is your best preventive medicine against any chronic eye problem.

- It can prevent any eye disorder.

- It can reverse any disorder you may already have developed.

- It can preserve and protect your remaining vision for the rest of your life.

Vision nutrition is your resource in self-healing. Prevention is always better than cure.

ANTIOXIDANTS

Vision nutrition is the most powerful weapon against free radicals, which are involved in the development of virtually all eye disorders, including cataracts, retinal disease, macular degeneration, and glaucoma, in the cellular level.

Antioxidants are powerful scavengers of free radicals in your body. They are substances in foods that disarm free radicals. Antioxidants include beta-carotene, coenzyme Q10, and vitamins A, C, and E.

The fluid that fills the front of your eye (known as *aqueous*) has one of the highest levels of vitamin C in your body. The retina at the back of your eye requires a good supply of antioxidant nutrients from your bloodstream.

Unfortunately, as you continue to age, your body produces fewer anti-oxidants, resulting in less protection of your eyes from oxidation.

In addition, the strong UV rays from the sun can burn or "oxidize" the retinal cells at the back you eyes, leading to loss of central vision. But lack of sunlight over many years can also destroy your retinal cells.

Foods to Fight Free Radicals

Foods that are rich in antioxidants are scavengers of free radicals.

- Chlorella is an alga containing high levels of chlorophyll (the green substance in plants). It is one of the purest and most potent foods on earth. Chlorella is a powerful detoxification agent against heavy metals and chemicals in your body. It not only breaks down persistent hydrocarbon and metallic toxins, such as mercury, cadmium, lead, DDT, and PCE, that you may have ingested in your body, but also strengthens your immune system.

- Eat several raw garlic cloves a day to fight free radicals. Overcome the odor by chewing some fresh parsley.

  A standard dosage of garlic is 900 mg daily of a garlic extract standardized to contain 1.3 percent *alliin*, the potent ingredient in garlic.

- Eat anti-aging foods high in vitamin C and bioflavonoids, such as apricots, berries, black currants, cherries, grapes, grapefruit, lemons, and plums, to prevent broken blood vessels and new blood vessel growth in the eye.

  Vitamin C does not stay in your body for long, so you need to replenish it constantly in order to reap its benefits.

- Load up on carrots for vitamin A. Carrots contain a *carotenoid* (a pigment in plants and animals that provides red and yellow color) called beta-carotene. Your body converts beta-carotene into vitamin A, which is a potent anti-oxidant for eye health and healthy vision. Eat carrots, and you will have eyes of an eagle.

- Protect the interior of your eyes from the sun with lutein (the primary carotenoid located in the center of the retina, called the macula) and zeaxanthin through supplements, or foods rich in lutein and zeaxanthin such as collard greens, Brussels sprouts, kale, green peas, pumpkin seeds, corn, green pepper, and spinach.

Cigarette smoking reduces the eye's production of lutein and zeaxanthin, which are pigments of the retina for filtering out harmful blue rays that thicken the macular pigment.

One cup of raw spinach contains about 18 mg. of lutein, one cup of cooked broccoli contains about 3 mg., and one cup of sliced green pepper around 1 mg. They are all anti-aging foods for vision health.

According to *The Journal of the American Medical Association* (JAMA), 5 servings of spinach per week may reduce macula degeneration by more than 50 percent.

- Take magnesium to aid blood flow to the eye for oxygen and nutrients.

- Consume cold-water fish and fish oils for omega-3 essential oils, as well as vitamins A and D, which aid in the production of protective pigments in the eye. Eating tuna may significantly reduce your dry eye symptoms.

- Take zinc to help release vitamin A from your liver to help healthy vision.

- Improve your night vision with bilberries, a cousin to blueberries, grown in the forest meadows of Europe, western Asia, and the northern Rocky Mountains. Bilberry is an herbal remedy that may have a very positive impact on night vision by fortifying blood vessel walls, thereby improving blood flow to the blood vessels in your eyes. Bilberry may help prevent macular degeneration and cataracts. Its original use traces back to World War II when British pilots found that eating jam made from bilberries helped them improve their night vision.

- Eat more protein (plant protein from beans) to reduce the development of cataracts, which make your eye's natural lens cloudy, according to a French scientific study.

- Supplement your diet with vitamin E from nuts to improve your healthy vision.

Balanced Acid-Alkaline to Combat Free Radicals

Your body cells need a balanced acid-and-alkaline environment to fight against free radicals. Acid and alkaline are substances that have opposing qualities. Your body functions at its best when the pH is optimum, which is slightly alkaline. The pH of your blood, tissues, and body fluids directly affect the state of your cellular health, in particular, that of the eye.

The pH scale ranges between one and fourteen. *Seven* is considered neutral. Anything *below* seven is considered *acidic*, while anything *above* seven is considered *alkaline*. Deviations above or below a 7.30 and 7.40 pH range can signal potentially serious and even dangerous symptoms, forewarning you of a disease in process.

When your body is too acidic, the tissues of your cells are forced to relinquish their alkaline reserves, depleting them of alkaline minerals, which are the components of the tissues themselves.

Over acidification comes from excess intake of foods containing great amounts of acid (animal proteins, sugar), and insufficient elimination by the body through the kidneys (urination) and the skin (sweating).

Alkaline foods contain little or no acid substances, and they do not produce acids when metabolized by your body. Alkaline foods include: green vegetables; colored vegetables (except tomato); chestnut; potato; avocado; black olives; bananas; dried fruits; almonds and Brazil nuts; alkaline mineral waters; cold-pressed oils (e.g. olive oil).

Alkaline medicinal plants also maintain the optimum pH level.

- Black currant fruits are a good source of vitamin C and other vitamins and minerals, including an omega-6 fatty acid to increase blood flow to the eye.

- Cranberry has been in use since the Iron Age, but the Romans were the first to recognize its medicinal values. Cranberry contains anti-asthmatic compounds, and is high in vitamin C and antioxidants. Eat fresh or dried cranberry, not the sugar-loaded cranberry juice obtainable in the supermarket.

Alkaline energy boosters can enhance your alkalinity to fight against free radicals.

- Blackstrap molasses is an excellent source of iron and calcium, copper, magnesium, manganese, and potassium.

  Make a healthy alkaline drink with a tablespoon of organic blackstrap molasses (mixed in some hot water first) and ¾ cup of soymilk. Add ice.

- Cod liver oil, which comes from fatty fish, such as salmon and sardines, is rich in vitamin A and vitamin D, and essential omega 3 oils. It enhances the absorption of calcium and maintains a constant level of blood calcium. Cod liver oil improves brain functions and the nervous system, which play a pivotal part in vision health.

Alkaline supplements, such as coral calcium, can keep all mineral levels up, and each and every mineral in balance. Alkaline supplements should contain calcium (Ca), sodium (Na), silica and copper, and other minerals to aid de-acidification of the body. More importantly, they should contain every mineral in similar proportion to that found in the human body. Remember, the human body functions synergistically: the whole is greater than the sum of its parts. Every mineral has its crucial role to play in the human anatomy, including the eye.

ESSENTIAL FATTY ACIDS

The high consumption of foods loaded with saturated fats and cholesterol, as well as man-made fats in egg substitutes, margarines, and basked foods, has led to a host of age-related eye disorders, such as macular degeneration, glaucoma, and retinal vein occlusion, among others. The explanation is that the tiny blood vessels located in the eye may become easily clogged with fats and other deposits that may cause eye problems.

The omega-3 fats, on the other hand, are good fats that help the normal functioning of the eye:

- Regulating eye pressur

- Moistening the eye

- Relieving spasms in the eyelids

- Reducing the eye's sensitivity to the sun

- Boosting the immune system

The omega-3 fats are found in chestnuts, flax seed, northern beans, soy, walnuts, wheat germ, and fish, such as cod, mackerel, salmon, and tuna.

For the omega-3 fats to be potent in protecting against free radicals, they must be combined with antioxidants.

THE LIVER HEALTH

For centuries, Oriental doctors have used the eye to diagnose different diseases: aching, bloodshot, bulging, itching, watery, and yellowish eyes reflect internal disharmony or disorder, in particular, that in the liver. Therefore, the liver health is also vision health.

The Importance of the Liver

The liver is called "liver" because it is a reflection of *how well* you have lived—essentially, your *lifestyle*. The liver is your main body organ responsible for distributing and maintaining your body's "fuel" supply.

According to Chinese medicine, the eyes are "the windows" of your internal health, especially that of your liver:

- Constant redness in the white of the eyes (dysfunctional circulatory and respiratory system)

- Yellowish skin under the eyes (overactive liver and gallbladder)

- Water-containing bags under the lower eyelids (congested digestive and excretory systems)

- Lack of luster (congested liver)

The Liver Functions

Therefore, the liver plays a pivotal part in your vision health. The liver serves several important functions in your body that may directly or indirectly affect your vision health:

- **Carbohydrate metabolism**

  The liver turns glucose (blood sugar) into glycogen (energy) for storage in your liver. Your glycogen controls the amount of glucose released into your bloodstream, thereby maintaining your blood sugar level. A healthy blood sugar levels prevents the development of diabetes, which impairs vision.

The liver regulates your carbohydrate metabolism, which plays an important role in your weight control.

- **Fat metabolism**

The liver is a fat-burning organ: it not only burns fat but also pumps excess fat out of your body system. Accordingly, your liver controls your body weight. Too much fat in the abdominal area may impair your fat metabolism, turning your liver into a "fatty liver" which then becomes a fat-storing organ. A "fatty liver" is an obstacle to any attempt at weight loss, which begins at the liver.

If you are obese, you have a much higher risk of losing your eyesight, according to the Royal National Institute for the Blind. For example, too much body fat is one of the causes of diabetes; too much fat may cause oxidative damage to the eye in macular degeneration.

- **Dietary cholesterol and toxin removal**

The liver detoxifies your body by filtering out excessive waste and toxins in your body through the bile into the gut. For example, it deactivates alcohol, hormones, and medicinal drugs for better assimilation.

Alcohol and certain pharmaceutical drugs have been implicated in vision loss. Always eat a high-fiber diet to facilitate elimination in order to prevent these toxic waste products from re-circulating back to your liver! In addition, chronic constipation may damage your liver, and thus your eyes.

- **Storage for nutrients**

    The liver stores glycogen, vitamins A and D, the B complex vitamins, iron and copper.

Apart from the brain, the liver is the most important body organ that affects your vision.

Liver Cleansing

A strong and healthy liver needs regular cleansing and detoxification. Here are some simple ways to regularly cleanse your liver:

- Drink organic unsweetened apple juice daily for 2 to 3 consecutive days to initiate liver detoxification.

- Eat a raw diet of only fruits and vegetables, with no dairy products, for 2 to 3 days.

- Drink a mixture of organic pure olive oil (4 ounces) and equal amount of fresh squeezed lemon juice. Shake well and drink immediately before going to bed.

- Drink ginger tea daily for liver and bowel cleansing: Juice one lemon, a two-inch fresh ginger root, four cloves, and one stick of cinnamon; add juice to two cups of water in a saucepan; bring to boil, and simmer for 10 - 15 minute; add a pinch of sea salt to your drinking water to alkalize it, as well as to provide important minerals and trace elements.

Enhancing Liver Health

A healthy liver filters approximately 3 pints of blood per minute, producing 1 to 1.5 quarts of bile daily.

A healthier liver gives you clear and sharp vision.

- **Eating raw**

  Eat some raw vegetables or drink fresh vegetable juice daily.

  A raw diet provides you with enzymes, which are required for optimum digestion and which are easily destroyed by heat during cooking.
  At least 20 to 30 percent of your diet should be raw fruits and vegetables.

- **Avoiding excess fat**

  Do not overload your liver and gall bladder with excess fatty foods, such as: animal milk (instead, drink rice milk and soymilk); foods with animal skins; deep-fried foods; full-cream dairy products; hydrogenated oils, and preserved meats

- **Consuming essential fatty acids**

  Essential fatty acids are fats in their natural, unprocessed form, such as: Alfalfa sprouts (you can easily grow alfalfa sprouts from seeds);

avocado; fish; flaxseed; pumpkin seeds; sesame seeds; and sunflower seeds

- **Eating proteins**

  Get non-animal proteins from the grains (brown rice and oatmeal), and raw seeds and nuts

  Eat animal proteins moderately, such as eggs from free-range chickens, and lean red meats

- **Eating healing foods for the liver**

  Eat beet, broccoli, cruciferous vegetables, garlic, ginger root, soy, and turmeric to help your liver detoxification. Include these healing foods in your diet as much as possible for optimum liver health!

- **Avoiding chemicals**

  Do not overload your liver with chemicals from supermarket foods and drinks, such as artificial sweeteners, Aspartame (in diet sodas), food colorings, food emulsifiers, and preservatives

  Always read food labels before any purchase! Go organic to eliminate pesticides and other chemicals!

- **Avoiding constipation**

  A bowel movement every other day is irregular, and a bowel movement once a day is still inadequate; a bowel movement twice or three times a day is optimum.

To optimize your elimination, do the following:

- o Eat a fiber-rich diet.

- o Eat fresh sweet corn raw, or only lightly cooked. Corn is an excellent blood-cleansing fiber.

- o Grind a handful of almonds, alfalfa seeds, flaxseeds, pumpkin seeds, sesame seeds, and sunflower seeds. Sprinkle them in your salads, soups, and smoothies.

- **Re-hydrating**

Re-hydrate your system with water and more fluids to avoid constipation and to enhance kidney elimination. Drink more than eight 8-oz glasses of water daily.

- **Intestinal hygiene**

Watch out for your intestinal hygiene.

- o Always eat fresh. Food poisoning is due to unfriendly bacteria and organisms put in a dormant state by food preservatives.

- o Do not reheat your food more than twice.

- o Do not eat while you are stressed: stress induces indigestion and bloating, because your blood flow is directed away from your intestines and liver.

- o Avoid fast foods and takeout foods as much as possible.

- o Always wash hands before preparing your food.

THE DIGESTIVE HEALTH

The incidence of eye disorders and diseases increases with age. Eye problems have been linked to *mal-absorption* of various nutrients needed for the eye due to an unhealthy digestive system.

- Dry eye syndrome: low levels of digestive juices

- Glaucoma: lack of absorption of thiamine (vitamin B1).

- Night vision problems: chronic liver disease (constipation)

- Red and irritated eyes: lack of digestive juices

The fact that eye problems are prevalent among the elderly population who also have digestive problems attests to the importance of the digestive health in healthy vision.

Your digestive system is one of the parts of your body that is often neglected. But good health begins on the inside.

Digestion is a complex process involving chemical and physical changes, such as breakdown of food and drinks into their small parts, absorption of nutrients by your body, conversion of food to energy for your body's use, and disposal of waste materials from your body. Your digestive tract is a long tube running from your mouth to your anus. Make this long tract clean and you will have healthy eyes.

The Digestion Process

The digestion process begins with your ingestion of food in your mouth. Your teeth and tongue break down or masticate food, and your salivary glands initiate chemical digestion by immediately secreting saliva with liquid enzymes to break down starches into sugar. Once the food is chewed and softened, your tongue rolls it into a ball, and then pushes it to the throat to be swallowed.

The food then passes into the esophagus, a muscular tube connecting the mouth with the stomach. The esophagus moves the food to the stomach by a series of muscular contractions.

When the food reaches your stomach, the gastric acid containing enzymes mixes with the food and begins mechanical digestion in which the food is churned to break down the proteins in your food. Proteins are the only substances digested in the stomach, but proteins are only partially digested in the stomach.

The undigested food then passes into your small intestine. Bile is released from your liver to prepare the digestion of fats, and pancreatic juice containing enzymes begins the digestion of carbohydrates, while the digestion of your partially digested proteins continues. In addition, the walls of your small intestine also release enzymes to complete the digestion in your small intestine.

Nutrients from your digested food is absorbed into blood vessels on the walls of your small intestine, and then carried to all your body cells and organs, including your eyes.

The material that has not been absorbed moves into the large intestine or colon. Here, water and salts are absorbed, and the remaining solid waste, converted to fecal matter, goes out of your body through the anus.

Incomplete Digestion

Incomplete digestion occurs when there is insufficient stomach acid to digest proteins, and inadequate pancreatic juice to digest fats and carbohydrates.

The presence of undigested food causes an overgrowth of unfriendly bacteria in the lower small intestine and in the colon. The toxins from these bacteria may begin to stress the liver, which has to work overtime to remove those toxins produced.

Efficient Digestion

Poor digestion may cause insomnia, which creates stress and strain for the eye. Therefore, efficient digestion should be encouraged. Improper dentures, over-sensitive teeth, and diseased gums may also affect your ability to chew your food adequately.

- Always chew your food thoroughly.

- Eat several smaller and lighter meals, instead of one or two heavy meals. As you grow older, reduced blood supply to your small intestine may adversely affect your capability to absorb nutrients from your food.

- Do not gulp liquids, or talk, while chewing food. Always eat in a *relaxed* manner—not watching the television or working on the computer. Be aware of the taste, texture of every morsel you put into your mouth.

- Eliminate dairy products from your diet, especially if you are allergic to them; avoid too much high-fat food.

- Avoid excessive eating when you are stressed.

- Avoid smoking and too much alcohol drinking, which may irritate your stomach lining.

- Eat a small piece of fresh ginger with lemon before a heavy meal to activate your salivary glands to produce enzymes to aid your digestion.

- Avoid cold drinks during a meal. Drink at least half an hour before or after, but not during, a meal.

- Do not lie down immediately after a meal; do not eat before you go to bed.

Learn to follow Nature's prescription of suitable times for your meals. Your lunch should be the heaviest meal, since your digestive fire is at its maximum potency. A late dinner interferes with your body's mechanism to detoxify and digest food from the day, making you tired the next morning you wake up. Most importantly, eat only when you are hungry, not necessarily because it is meal time.

Enhancing Digestive Health

- **Colon cleansing**

  Colon cleansing is a must for a healthy digestive system and healthy vision.

  - Add one teaspoon of **Epsom salts** (magnesium sulfate) to one glass of water. Drink this first thing in the morning for up to three weeks. Do this treatment at least twice a year.

  - Alternatively, take one to three teaspoons of **Castor oil** in a glass of warm water. Drink it the first thing in the morning or on an empty stomach before going to bed. Do this treatment on a regular basis, or as often as needed.

- **Kidney cleansing**

  Check to see if you may have kidney stones by pulling the skin under your eyes sideways toward your cheekbones to see if there is any visible pimple or protrusion, or discoloration of the skin.

- **Fasting to detoxify**

Go on water fast at least once a month to detoxify your body of accumulated toxins. Drink only water with no food.

- **Drinking enough water**

  Drink enough water to maintain adequate bile production and bile consistency.

LIFESTYLE CHANGES

Impaired vision is one of the major causes of frailty of old age. Your vision is important to you. The rest of your life, your welfare and your well-being depend upon good eyesight. Maintaining healthy vision goes a long way to prolonging your ability to function fully in life further down the road.

To keep your eyes healthier and for longer, you may have to make some lifestyle changes:

Alcohol

Alcohol addiction may lead to the development of alcoholic liver disease (ALD), which causes irreparable liver damage, and thus adversely affecting vision. ALD comes in three stages:

- **The fatty liver stage**

  At this stage, the liver demonstrates abnormalities but without evident signs of deterioration. With abstinence from alcohol, the abnormal conditions of the fatty liver are reversible.

- **The alcoholic hepatitis stage**

  At this stage, the liver functions become abnormal and irregular, with the development of **jaundice**, which is indicated by yellowish coloring of the eyes and the skin. The conditions may still be reversible with complete abstinence from alcohol.

- **The cirrhosis stage**

  This is the final and irreversible stage of ALD. The liver becomes scarred, with the development of liver nodules, jaundice, and bleeding. At this stage, vision is greatly impaired.
  Prevention is always better than cure. Cirrhosis is preventable with the abstinence of alcohol.
  In its early stages, alcoholic liver disease (ALD) can be significantly improved with the following:

  - An antioxidant-rich diet, high in vitamin E and selenium.

  - A normal body weight

  - Nutritional supplements to compensate for loss of nutrients due to loss of appetite and nausea, which are common conditions of alcoholic liver disease

Don't drink too much alcohol! If you have a drinking problem, learn to give up alcohol addiction.

Nicotine

Cigarette smoke impairs vision.

- The tar in cigarette smoke is composed of chemicals, poisons, and corrosives, such as hydrogen cyanide and carbon monoxide, which deprive your heart and your eyes of essential oxygen for optimum functioning.

- Cigarette smoke produces free radicals that destroy eye tissues.

- Smoking damages the heart, responsible for transporting oxygen and nutrients to the eye, and the nervous system. Nicotine, which is a poison in itself, damages the nervous system, which is directly connected with vision.

- Smoking not only restricts blood flow to the eye, but also promotes the deposits of fat and cholesterol that may clog the blood vessels in the eye, leading to the development of eye problems.

- Smokers tend to develop early cataracts or have early onset of glaucoma.

- Smokers often have a tendency to wrinkle and pucker their eyelids, causing unnecessary eyestrain.

Quitting the habit may not be easy, especially if smoking has already become a habit or an addiction. Nearly 80 percent of smokers who strive to kick the habit will suffer relapses and experience the following withdrawal symptoms:

- Slowing down of heart rate

- Elevation of blood pressure

- Development of ulcers

- Lack of mental concentration

- Anxiety and depression

- Drowsiness

- Gastrointestinal disturbances

Quitting may therefore put you in a catch-22 situation. However, the long-term effects of smoking on vision are disastrous and far-reaching. Quit smoking at all costs. Success in quitting is contingent upon the following:

- You must make the personal decision to quit smoking to keep your eyes healthier for longer. Nobody can make that decision for you. Only you can decide to quit.

- You must overcome the denial that smoking is a systematic suicide. This initiates your desire to make the decision to quit.

- You must persist and persevere in taking repeated actions to quit smoking, despite repeated relapses and failures. Remember, **Sir**

Winston Churchill once said: "Never, never, never give up!" You must also do the same— never, never, never give up quitting smoking!

You must make a commitment to take the necessary actions, and success will be the follow-through.

APPENDIX A

GOOD VISION HABITS

Good vision habits involve developing good habits of the body, the mind, and the eye.

PHYSICAL HABITS

Develop **good posture** to provide good blood circulation to the brain and to the visual system. Nearsighted people usually have tension in upper back, shoulders, neck, and around the eyes, resulting from poor posture.

- Sit upright to read at eye level to avoid straining the eye, the neck and shoulder muscles.

- Sit with your pelvis back in the seat, and your feet on the floor. Do not slouch, sag or curve your shoulders. Sitting is hard on your lower back. Your sitting posture is as important as your standing posture to your overall posture health. Good posture means sitting properly:

- o **Sit with *neutral* pelvis** (pelvis not tilting forward).

- o Do not lean over a desk (head-forward position), putting undue pressure on your neck and upper back.

- o Do not rest against the back.

- o Lift your rib cage.

- o Press your belly button into your spine.

- o Stick your chin forward and pull back your head and neck.

- o Keep your head high and flatten your upper back.

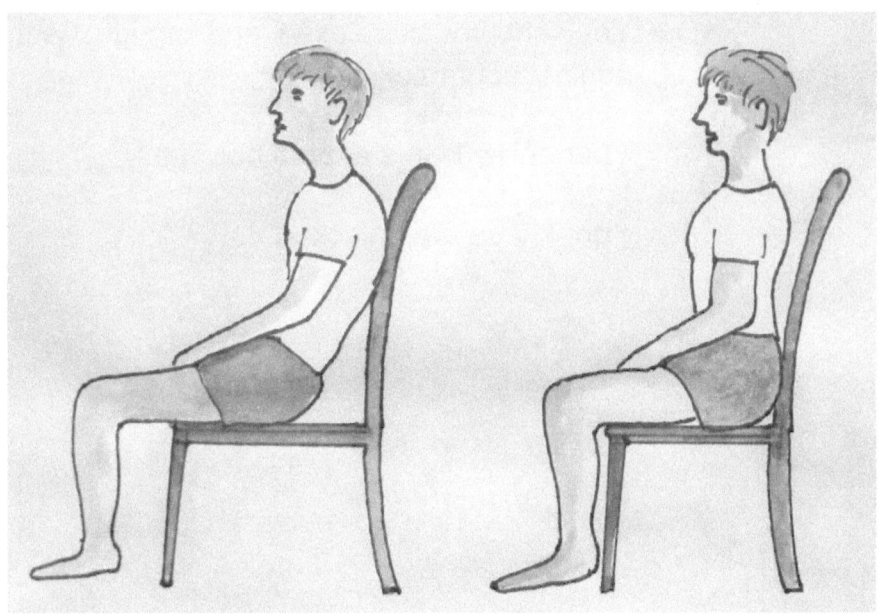

Incorrect sitting position   Correct sitting position

- **Stand erect** to attain even distribution of body weight for body relaxation. Good posture means in any standing position, you body posture should be as follows:

    o   Stand tall with your chin and tummy tucked in.

    o   Your head is directly above your shoulders.

    o   Your ear, shoulder, and hip are in a straight line from a side view.

    o   Your upper back is straight, not slouched.

o Your shoulders, relaxed and straight, are flat against your back.

o Your pelvis is in a neutral position.

o Your knees are unlocked.

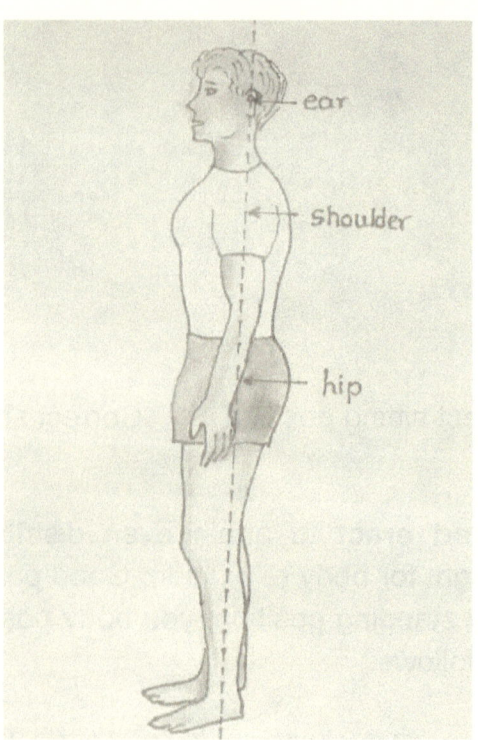

Exercise to enhance good standing posture

o Stand with your back against a wall with heels

o several inches away from the wall.

o Relax your arms.

- o Slowly bend your knees, while pressing the small of your back against the wall.
- o Lift your rib cage and press the back of your head to the wall.

- o Press the back of your shoulders to the wall,

- o while pulling the shoulder blades together.

- o Hold the position.

- o Press your back and shoulders to the wall.

- o Bend your knees and slide down the wall.

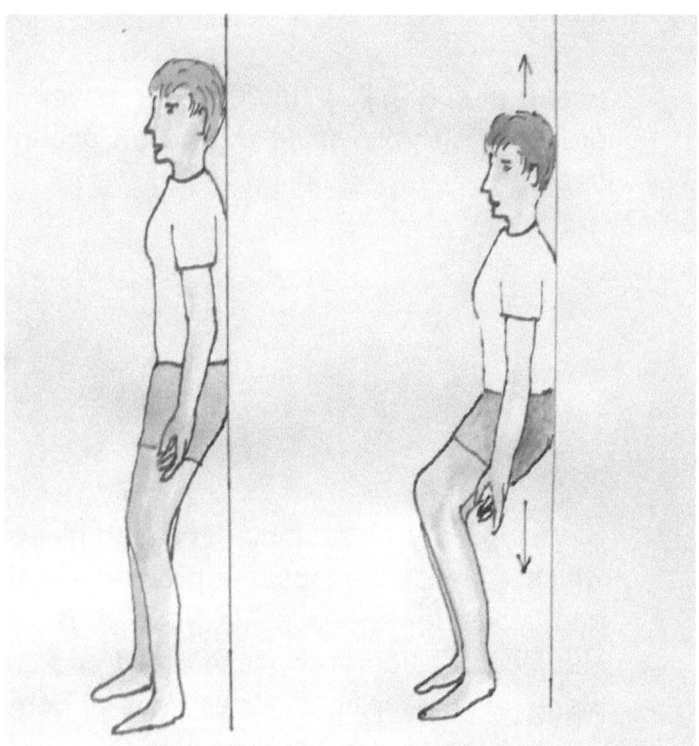

- **Sleep on the side** with a small pillow between legs to

relax the spine, which controls the trunk, the neck, and the head, and hence the eye.

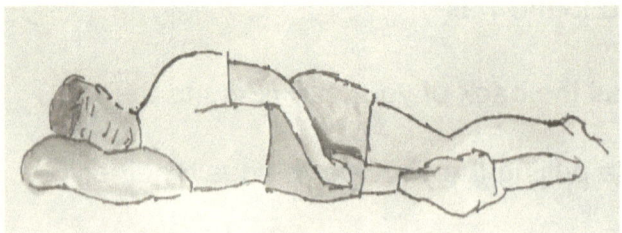

Sleeping on your back is not an ideal sleeping position. However, if you are accustomed to this sleeping position, then sleep on a thin pillow—head leveling with your spine. Avoid pushing your head forward or arching your neck with your chin jutting forward.

Place a soft pillow under your lower legs to take pressure off your spine due to an accentuated lower back.

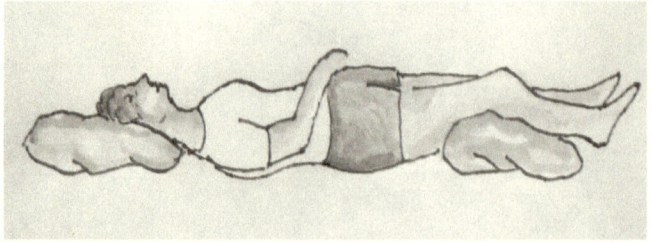

Sleeping on your stomach is a bad sleeping position, which may cause posture problems with your neck and your lower back. If your must assume this sleeping position, sleep with a soft and flat pillow, and place a small pillow under your abdomen to avoid sagging your lower back.

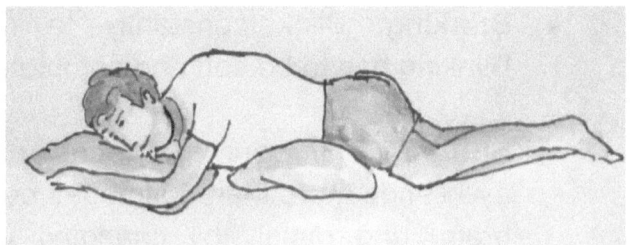

If possible, learn to change your sleeping position.
A good sleeping position induces natural sleep for
deep body and mental relaxation.

MENTAL HABITS

- Make no comparison between vision without
  glasses and vision with glasses. Learn to be
  comfortable with blur. Do not strive to see clearly.
  Clear vision will automatically come with improved
  vision.

- Clear vision has to do with the strength of the eye
  muscles, and the shape of the eye. Mind power
  has this capability.

- Harness your mind power for self-affirmations and
  positive visualization for vision improvement.

VISUAL HABITS

Develop good visual habits to enhance your vision
improvement.

- **Blinking**: Blink constantly to relax the eye. Blinking has to be soft and complete, not rapid.

- **Shifting**: Shift your eyes constantly (the healthy eye sends more than 50 images per second to the brain) and rapidly by changing your eye focus frequently. Your eyes move more rapidly when they are relaxed.

- **Peripheral vision**: Be aware of your total field of vision whenever you focus your eyes. Use BOTH central vision and peripheral vision at the same time.

- **Natural sunlight**: Spend more time outdoors instead of indoors to reap the health benefits of sunlight in nourishing your visual system.

- **Palming**: Relaxation of the eye cures all vision problems. The eye rests completely only in total darkness. Practice palming and visualize blackness even for as little as 1 to 2 minutes per session. Of course, the longer you palm, the more relaxed your eyes become.

- **Vision without glasses**: See without glasses to bring back your eye's natural "accommodation" for better vision. However, remember not to strain to see without glasses. Reduce your time of wearing glasses, and delay the time you put on glasses in the morning. Use under-corrected prescription to slowly and gradually wean yourself from wearing corrective lenses.

VISION AWARENESS

Vision health is all about **awareness**—awareness of what you should do and what you should not do. Your conscious mind may want to change the bad vision habits that continue to impair your vision, but it is constantly held back by your subconscious mind.

Form the habit of awareness. Always be aware of the following good vision habits:

- To heal the eye, *change* your vision habits!

- Your mind determines how your eyes see!

- Use your subconscious mind to change your vision with affirmations and visualization!

- Breathe right to relax both the body and the mind!

- Consciously train your eyes for distant vision! Regularly look up from your computer or your book!

- The shape of the eyeball determines the power of vision. The relaxation level of the eye pre-determines the shape of the eyeball!

- See only *selectively*! Never STRAIN your eyes to see! A blurry image is OK!

- Not need to go for perfect vision! Never STRAIN your eyes in order to see better!

- Look without blinking (soft vision) for 10

seconds or so!

- Do not stare! Blink to stop frozen gaze!

- Do not let a day pass by without palming your eyes!

- Always blink—soft and complete! Form the habit of constant blinking!

- Train your eyes for peripheral vision to see what is on both sides of your eyes!

- Swing and shift for clear and soft vision!

- Edge and track anytime and anywhere!

APPENDIX B

SIGNS OF VISION IMPROVEMENT

Your visual improvement will not only take time but also undergo different stages of changes.

Physical Signs of Vision Improvement

The physical signs of improvement may include:

- Eyes becoming more relaxed, feeling less tense

- Black becoming blacker

- Colors becoming more vibrant

- Brief moments of clearer and wider vision

- Less sensitivity to sunlight, and easier adaptation from light to darkness, and vice-versa.

Mental Signs of Vision Improvement

The mental signs of vision improvement may include:

- More mental energy

- Sharper mental focus, including greater concentration

- More creative and imaginative

- Better memory

Symptoms of Vision Readjustment

Your eye conditions may undergo a period of *readjustment* before ultimate vision improvement occurs, and these temporary symptoms may include eye tiredness, headaches, watery eyes, and changes in balance and orientation

Natural vision improvement takes time. Remember the following:

- You must get yourself accustomed to blurry vision around you as a result of not wearing eyeglasses or contacts.
- You must not strain to see clearly when your vision is blurry.

- You will see clearly when your vision improves.

APPENDIX C

COMPUTER VISUAL STRESS

Using computers is a way of life, and only few of us can do without a computer in our daily lives.

Using **video display terminals** (VDTs) on a regular basis will inevitably lead to computer visual stress. Prolonged VDT use causes two common eye problems: **focusing** and **eye coordination**. Other side effects may include: headaches, blurring of images, and eyestrain.

Computer visual stress takes a great toll on the eye with respect to the following:

- **Binocularity** (using both eyes together)

- **Convergence** (bringing the eyes together at close range)

- **Eye accommodation** (focusing)

- **Shifting** (eye movement skill)

Computer-induced visual stress is a common workplace problem, which is manifested in nearsightedness, eyestrain, eye focusing difficulties, changes in color perception, double vision, and general stress.

Optimizing the Computer System

Be aware of how information appears on your computer screen, and adjust your tracking and scanning visual skills accordingly.

- The characters on your computer screen should be 10 times brighter than the screen background.

- The lighting of the room should be three times brighter than the computer screen background.

- The character size should be appropriate: approximately 80 characters per line with 25 lines per screen.

- The VDT viewing distance (18 – 25 inches) should be greater than the normal reading distance (12 – 16 inches). The recommended viewing distance is 20 inches between the eye and the computer screen.

- The line of sight to the top of the computer should be 20 degrees below horizontal, and the line of sight to the bottom of the screen should be 20 degrees lower.

Overcoming Computer-Induced Visual Stress

The following are some of the tips to reduce or overcome computer-induced visual stress:

- Use a **screen filter** to help eliminate the glare, static, and radiation problems related with VDT viewing.

- Every now and then, rotate your head forward and backward, and sideways to relieve tension in the neck, which may adversely affect the functioning of the eye.

- Do the **palming exercise** to relax the eye; even a 2-minute session will significantly relieve eyestrain.

- Do the **thumb rotation exercise**:

    o Sit in a relaxed posture.

    o Cover your right eye with your right hand.

    o Hold out the left hand directly in front of your nose, with your elbow straight. Slightly clench your fingers, leaving the thumb erect.

    o Now, look at your thumbnail, and begin moving your left arm up, then outward and downward to a point that is level with your nose (like in a quarter circle).

    o Follow your thumbnail with your left eye. Move only your arm and your eyeball.

○   Repeat the above with your right hand

The objective of this thumb rotation exercise is to improve your eye movement and to organize your visual space. You can easily practice this exercise even at your workplace

Given that computer-induced visual stress may have long-term impact on your vision health, be aware of the time you spend on the computer. It is very important to give yourself breaks and during those breaks, give yourself time to practice eye palming exercise to relax your eyes. Remember, even a five-minute palming will do wonders to relax your eyes.

APPENDIX D

VISION IMPROVEMENT IMAGES

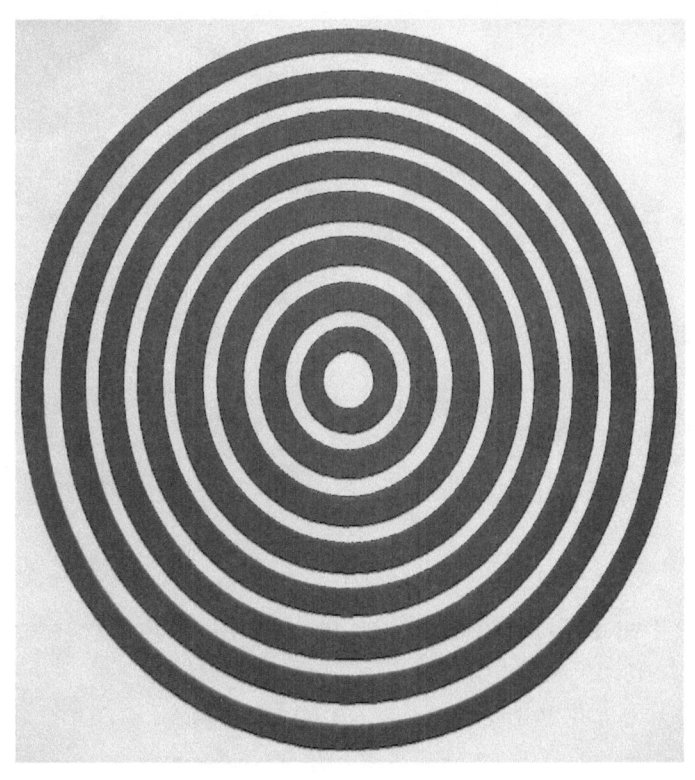

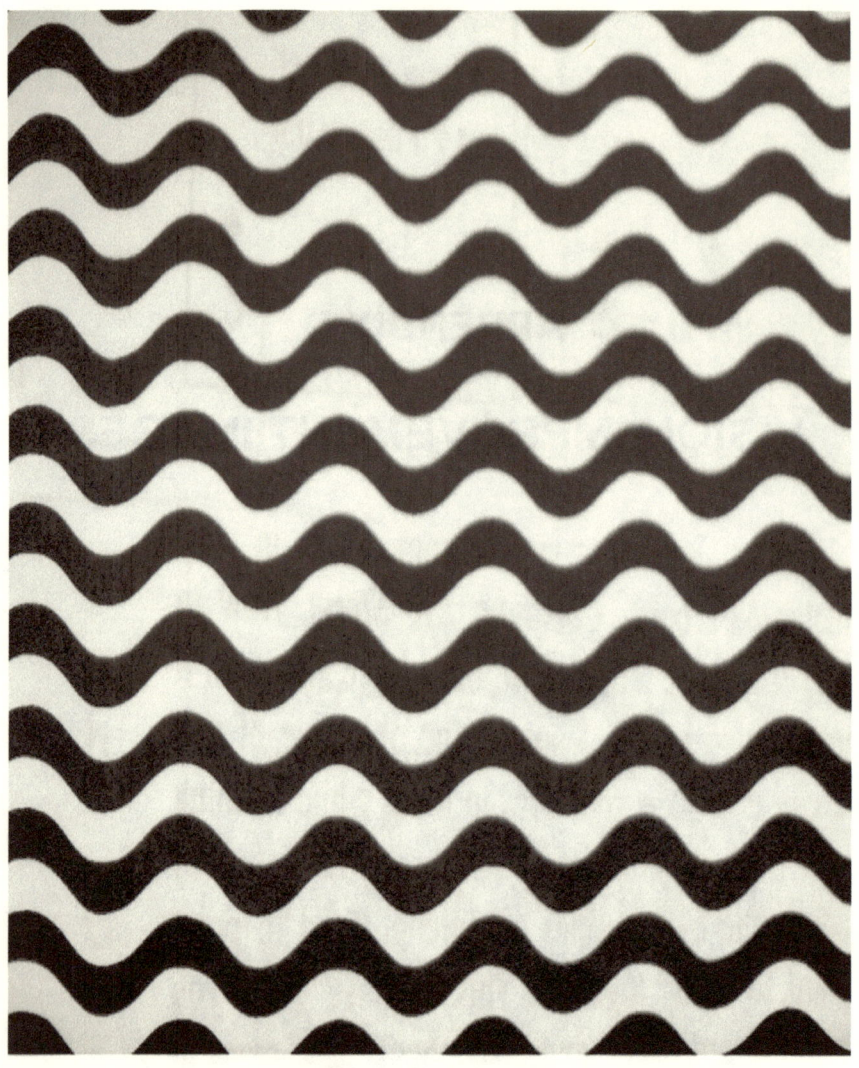

Use the above images to train your eyes to see whole fields of vision all at once.

Use the following eye charts to train your vision

A C G B

F M 8 J O P K

X Q N 2 U D

T L Y 9 4 V F 7 A M 3

D R W 3 T 8 K L M

Make use of the charts and images to train your eyes for better vision

Final words of wisdom: vision self-healing is a reality, not a myth. Believe in yourself that you can make your eyes better than what they are right now. Practice vision awareness and eye exercises and relaxation techniques,

Good luck and God bless you!

Stephen Lau.

ABOUT STEPHEN LAU

Stephen Lau is a writer and researcher who has book publications on wisdom in living, health and wellness, and ESL learning.

To find out more, visit his website: **All About Stephen Lau**: http://www.stephencmlau.com

Also, visit his **blogs**:

- **Increase Mind Power**
  http://www.increase-mind-power.blogspot.com

- **Myasthenia Gravis Disorder**
  http://www.myasthenia-gravis-disorder.blogspot.com

- **Natural Health Wisdom**
  http://www.natural-health-wisdom.com

- **Reflections of Stephen Lau**
  http://www.reflectionsofstephenlau.blogspot.com

- **Self-Healing-Resources**
  http://www.self-healing-resources.blogspot.com

- **Tao Wisdom for All**:
  http://www.tao-wisdom-for-all.blogspot.com

- **BLOG for ESL**
  http://www.blog-for-esl.blog.com

- **Effective Writing Made Simple**
  http://www.effective-writing-made-simple.blogspot.com

Also, subscribe to his **Wellness Wisdom Newsletter**: http://www.wellness-wisdom-newsletter.com